Marek R. Ogiela, Ryszard Tadeusiewicz

Modern Computational Intelligence Methods for the Interpretation of Medical Images

Studies in Computational Intelligence, Volume 84

Editor-in-chief
Prof. Janusz Kacprzyk
Systems Research Institute
Polish Academy of Sciences
ul. Newelska 6
01-447 Warsaw
Poland
E-mail: kacprzyk@ibspan.waw.pl

Further volumes of this series
can be found on our homepage:
springer.com

Vol. 60. Vladimir G. Ivancevic and Tijana T. Ivacevic
Computational Mind: A Complex Dynamics Perspective, 2007
ISBN 978-3-540-71465-1

Vol. 61. Jacques Teller, John R. Lee and Catherine Roussey (Eds.)
Ontologies for Urban Development, 2007
ISBN 978-3-540-71975-5

Vol. 62. Lakhmi C. Jain, Raymond A. Tedman and Debra K. Tedman (Eds.)
Evolution of Teaching and Learning Paradigms in Intelligent Environment, 2007
ISBN 978-3-540-71973-1

Vol. 63. Wlodzislaw Duch and Jacek Mańdziuk (Eds.)
Challenges for Computational Intelligence, 2007
ISBN 978-3-540-71983-0

Vol. 64. Lorenzo Magnani and Ping Li (Eds.)
Model-Based Reasoning in Science, Technology, and Medicine, 2007
ISBN 978-3-540-71985-4

Vol. 65. S. Vaidya, L.C. Jain and H. Yoshida (Eds.)
Advanced Computational Intelligence Paradigms in Healthcare-2, 2007
ISBN 978-3-540-72374-5

Vol. 66. Lakhmi C. Jain, Vasile Palade and Dipti Srinivasan (Eds.)
Advances in Evolutionary Computing for System Design, 2007
ISBN 978-3-540-72376-9

Vol. 67. Vassilis G. Kaburlasos and Gerhard X. Ritter (Eds.)
Computational Intelligence Based on Lattice Theory, 2007
ISBN 978-3-540-72686-9

Vol. 68. Cipriano Galindo, Juan-Antonio Fernández-Madrigal and Javier Gonzalez
A Multi-Hierarchical Symbolic Model of the Environment for Improving Mobile Robot Operation, 2007
ISBN 978-3-540-72688-3

Vol. 69. Falko Dressler and Iacopo Carreras (Eds.)
Advances in Biologically Inspired Information Systems: Models, Methods, and Tools, 2007
ISBN 978-3-540-72692-0

Vol. 70. Javaan Singh Chahl, Lakhmi C. Jain, Akiko Mizutani and Mika Sato-Ilic (Eds.)
Innovations in Intelligent Machines-1, 2007
ISBN 978-3-540-72695-1

Vol. 71. Norio Baba, Lakhmi C. Jain and Hisashi Handa (Eds.)
Advanced Intelligent Paradigms in Computer Games, 2007
ISBN 978-3-540-72704-0

Vol. 72. Raymond S.T. Lee and Vincenzo Loia (Eds.)
Computation Intelligence for Agent-based Systems, 2007
ISBN 978-3-540-73175-7

Vol. 73. Petra Perner (Ed.)
Case-Based Reasoning on Images and Signals, 2008
ISBN 978-3-540-73178-8

Vol. 74. Robert Schaefer
Foundation of Global Genetic Optimization, 2007
ISBN 978-3-540-73191-7

Vol. 75. Crina Grosan, Ajith Abraham and Hisao Ishibuchi (Eds.)
Hybrid Evolutionary Algorithms, 2007
ISBN 978-3-540-73296-9

Vol. 76. Subhas Chandra Mukhopadhyay and Gourab Sen Gupta (Eds.)
Autonomous Robots and Agents, 2007
ISBN 978-3-540-73423-9

Vol. 77. Barbara Hammer and Pascal Hitzler (Eds.)
Perspectives of Neural-Symbolic Integration, 2007
ISBN 978-3-540-73953-1

Vol. 78. Costin Badica and Marcin Paprzycki (Eds.)
Intelligent and Distributed Computing, 2008
ISBN 978-3-540-74929-5

Vol. 79. Xing Cai and T.-C. Jim Yeh (Eds.)
Quantitative Information Fusion for Hydrological Sciences, 2008
ISBN 978-3-540-75383-4

Vol. 80. Joachim Diederich
Rule Extraction from Support Vector Machines, 2008
ISBN 978-3-540-75389-6

Vol. 81. K. Sridharan
Robotic Exploration and Landmark Determination, 2008
ISBN 978-3-540-75393-3

Vol. 82. Ajith Abraham, Crina Grosan and Witold Pedrycz (Eds.)
Engineering Evolutionary Intelligent Systems, 2008
ISBN 978-3-540-75395-7

Vol. 83. Bhanu Prasad and S.R.M. Prasanna (Eds.)
Speech, Audio, Image and Biomedical Signal Processing using Neural Networks, 2008
ISBN 978-3-540-75397-1

Vol. 84. Marek R. Ogiela and Ryszard Tadeusiewicz
Modern Computational Intelligence Methods for the Interpretation of Medical Images, 2008
ISBN 978-3-540-75399-5

Marek R. Ogiela
Ryszard Tadeusiewicz

Modern Computational Intelligence Methods for the Interpretation of Medical Images

With 168 Figures and 3 Tables

Springer

Prof. Dr. Marek R. Ogiela
Prof. Dr. Ryszard Tadeusiewicz

Department of Bio Cybernetics
AGH University of Science and Technology
Kraków
Poland
mogiela@agh.edu.pl, rtad@agh.edu.pl

ISBN 978-3-642-44636-8 ISBN 978-3-540-75402-2 (eBook)

Studies in Computational Intelligence ISSN 1860-949X

Softcover re-print of the Hardcover 1st edition 2008

Cover Design: Deblik, Berlin, Germany

Printed on acid-free paper

9 8 7 6 5 4 3 2 1

springer.com

Contents

1. Introduction

The book presents just a small part of the huge body of knowledge which the authors use almost every day in their work on medical images [30–44, 54–61]. Not all the methods, algorithms and techniques presented in the book were developed by the authors themselves, but most them were applied to practical medical problems, some were improved and sometimes also devised in more than a decade of the authors' research on the processing, analyzing, classifying, recognizing and automatically interpreting medical images (and other data).

Those readers who professionally examine visual data (especially in clinical applications) or are experienced in using computer vision software can skip or omit the next three chapters. All other readers are strongly recommended to read the initial part of the book very carefully, as it presents the background and an introduction to the subject of computer image analysis.

Chapter 2 describes the basics of medical data acquisition methods. It is very short compared to the majority of books which describe the relevant technologies used for medical imaging in detail. The reason is that this book is focuses on image analysis and recognition and not acquisition and processing. Nevertheless, the unique properties of medical images are very much the product of the specific processes of their acquisition, so anyone wanting to use a computer for medical data analysis must know how those medical images are produced, at least in very general terms. Such a brief "all you need to know" is given in chapter 2.

Chapter 3 is an attempt at discussing the key factors of medical image compression problems. Due to the large sizes of state-of-the-art medical images combined with the rapidly growing number of imaging results obtained during the examination of every single patient, medical images need compressing if we want to save them to mass storage or send them from one computer to another (sometimes halfway around the world). But, we evidently cannot accept any image processing method that would result in losing information important from the diagnostic or therapeutic point of view.

It has already been mentioned that one of the most important features of medical images is their huge volume of information they contain. Everybody apparently realizes this, but in fact the actual scale of the problem can be unimaginable to a typical user of medical images. Let us calculate the data volume of a typical result of – for example – a CT examination. Let us assume image dimensions of 4096 times 4096 pixels with the resolution of 2 bytes per pixel. Let us further assume 20 slides (results of sequential scans) per examination. The resulting volume of information is 335,544,320 bytes. Now let us assess the volume of this information. One typical page of text is equal to approximately 2 Kb of information. One book (like this one) of 200 pages (excluding figures) represents 400 Kb of information. That means that the images representing the results of one medical examination of one patient are equivalent to more than 800 books. That is a really big library!

M.R. Ogiela and R. Tadeusiewicz: *Introduction,* Studies in Computational Intelligence (SCI) **84**, 1–6 (2007)
www.springerlink.com

This huge volume of information must be stored in medical records. It can be calculated that the total amount of information to be stored in a typical hospital database increases at the rate of over 10^{16} bites annually. Even with the biggest magnetic and optical disks and other database hardware, storage space must be conserved somehow.

The most effective method of storage space saving is data compression, so we must consider methods used for compressing images. There are many image compression algorithms, but not all of them can be used to compress medical images. This is because of the special demands due to the specific role of medical images, quite different from the role of many other images. If we are dealing with images to be used as figures in books or articles, a good legibility of the image after one compression-decompression cycle is sufficient to qualify the lossy compression algorithm used as acceptable. Even if some details of the original image are lost, the general impression that the reader gets is good so even very "aggressive" lossy methods of compression providing a high compression rate (evaluated as the gain in terms of the relation between the volume of the image before and after compression) can be used for this purpose, even if the quality of the resulting image is not very high.

On the contrary, a medical image should commands more respect. If the image will form the basis of diagnostic reasoning, and if such a diagnosis can make the difference between the life and death of a human being, then every minute detail becomes crucial. Nobody can give a general assurance that a lossy method of compression is "safe enough" because the removed (lost) details of the image are worthless. Consequently, we must primarily consider lossless methods of compression for medical imaging purposes. Unfortunately, such methods are not very effective and therefore we must sometimes also use lossy methods of image compression, but due care and controls.

The problems of medical image compression are presented and discussed in chapter 3.

Chapter 4 summarizes key properties of medical images which must be taken into account during all processes of their computer preparation, evaluation and interpretation. It would seem that all generally known methods of signal processing (e.g. filtration) can by used without any limitation for medical images. But in fact, some of those methods can be used for images, particularly for medical ones, while others cannot. The reason is very similar as in the case of image compression discussed above. Sometimes, de-noising a medical image can aid its interpretation by a physician or by automatic analytical procedures, but it can often be dangerous, as important and useful features of the medical image can be removed along with the noise.

We must once again emphasize that medical images need not be nice or pretty – they must be legible in terms of medical diagnostics. Typical image processing methods used for image enhancement in computer vision yield output images which look better than the input ones. Looked at as a whole, the image is very nice. But in the case of medical images, we do not look at the whole picture. On the contrary, we focus on particular elements or on selected features. Consequently, some image processing methods are useless for medical images, because the pretty images produced by advanced filtering procedures are worse than source images. Many examples can be shown where popular filtering procedures hide all the diagnostic information present in the source image together with most of the noise.

These specific features of medical images, stemming from their special purpose and the specific methods of their acquisition, are presented and discussed in chapter 4.

Chapter 5 presents multiple methods of image handling which can be used for medical data processing, obviously taking into account the limitations described above. Readers of this chapter must differentiate between two contexts:

The first and (so far) most typical context is the traditional way of "manual" image-based medical diagnosis (or therapy planning). In this first context we need only extract from the human body a good image of the organ to be analyzed, remove the noise, enhance features and give the prepared image to the doctor, who will make the decision. In the course of image processing performed under these presumptions we must take into account the perceptional limitations of the human eye, but we can also hope that the interpretation will be done in the most intelligent way possible. This in particular means that we can not show images with more than approximately 60 different levels of signal intensity (gray levels) to the doctor for him to make the recognition, because 60 is the maximum number of different gray levels perceivable by humans. However, the way in which key features of the diseased organ are presented in the image to be analyzed can be very complicated, as the human brain can discover even the most complex differentiation rules.

The second context to be considered when planning the preprocessing applies if image processing is followed by the automatic analysis of image features during which we try to automatically classify or understand the images. In this context, the number of features taken into account at the same time can be very big and the distance between the minimum and maximum values of every parameter can be practically unlimited. Unfortunately, this goes hand in hand with the requirement for relatively simple and known rules for differentiation between e.g. the ill and the healthy organ, or its discovery must be available in an a priori determined way (for example by the learning of a decision tree, support vector machines or neural networks).

The general purpose methods of image processing described and discussed in chapter 4 are supplemented by a dedicated method of medical image processing presented in chapter 5. In more than fifteen years of hard research work on many kinds of medical images, with many algorithms used for decision-making processes in medical diagnostics, the authors of this book have tried to develop many special methods for medical image processing. These special methods can be used for special-purpose medical image processing, because they were designed for the **automatic understanding** of such images. These methods can also be suitable for both manual decision-making processes and for the automatic recognition. selected results of such original investigations are presented in chapter 5.

All methods used for medical image processing, described in chapters 4 and 5 can generally be referred to as transformations leading from one image to another. In fact, all of them can be considered to be algorithms working with images on both the input and the output. This kind of processing can change the quality of the image, but cannot yield any useful, new information. If something can be seen in the image (for example symptoms of an illness), then after proper processing it can be seen more clearly and precisely on the image. Sometimes, in fact very often, the physician needs more help from the computer analyzing the image. For precise diagnostic examinations, we must have more information, that is more than the information available by means of a general perusal of the image. Such new information can be generated on the basis of a medical image if and only if we subject the image to analysis instead of processing. During the analysis, we can divide the image into a collection of separate elements (objects). Every element can then be described separately by means of many parameters relating to, respectively, its form (shape) or texture.

There are many image analysis methods described in computer vision theory and there are many goals relating in terms of the parameters and image features encountered during the analysis, but only some of them can be used to analyze medical images. These problems are described and discussed in chapter 6.

Medical image features that can be analyzed are either quantitative or qualitative. Quantitative parameters assessed during image analysis mostly represent the results of various measurements made in the digital image. In fact, the measurement process is based on computer calculations instead of surveying with special devices, nevertheless the result of the calculation is numerical. Another type are parameters connected with some qualitative evaluation of selected features of the image. For example, brain images considered to be healthy or pathological are typically tested using symmetry criteria. The brain in a real image in never ideally symmetrical in the way that a mathematical figure is. But if the asymmetry is major, it can form a important sign of pathology. Asymmetry cannot be expressed as an exactly measured value, but it can be described as a qualitative parameter with the values of: *symmetry, small asymmetry, average asymmetry, major asymmetry.*

Selected problems of medical image analysis processes as well as the types of quantitative and qualitative parameters encountered during these processes are presented in chapter 6.

After the image has been analyzed, there are several parameters describing and characterizing the objects and other elements visible in it, but this is only halfway to the conclusions needed by doctors. Even a great number of very sophisticated parameters cannot help the physician in diagnostic examinations if he/she cannot build a proper model of the decision making process leading from such parameters to the recognition of disease symptoms in his/her mind.

Fortunately, such a decision making process can also be computer-aided by applying modern pattern recognition methods. Descriptions of some pattern recognition methods and their applications are also discussed in chapter 6.

The sequence beginning with acquiring medical images, through their filtering and other processing stages, followed by the analysis and evaluation of their features and parameters and ending in the automatic classification and recognition methods represents the traditional sequence. It has been described in many books and developed in many a research project. Therefore the first 6 chapters of the book are not very original, although useful. The ultimate chapters – 7 and 8 – are a completely different story.

Chapter 7 proposes, presented, develops, discusses, and evaluates the original, new idea of the **automatic understanding of medical images**. The authors propose automatic understanding as the next step in the sequence of medical image acquisition, processing etc., after pattern recognition. Automatic understanding methods at-attempt at discovering the substantive content of the image in a way similar to that taking place in the physician's mind when he/she thinks about the medical image (and not just looks at it). Medical image understanding gives us the semantic meaning of the image, what can be extremely useful in many cases where simple image analysis and recognition is not enough.

In chapter 8, this new idea of automatic understanding is applied to two kinds of complex medical images. The first to be analyzed are images of wrist bones in which we must not only account for the shapes and dimensions of particular objects (palm bones), but also extract diagnostic information hidden in spatial relations between these objects. The second example is the application of the structural analysis and automatic understanding technology to the evaluation of 3D coronary artery images.

We hope that this book will help you come up with many useful, successful applications of computer vision methods to various types of medical images.

To conclude this introduction we should emphasize that the subject of this publication, i.e. the problems and methods of computational intelligence and their suitability for the in-depth analysis of medical images, focuses on the very important topic of techniques for the automatic understanding of such images. This is the main advantage of this publication, which the authors have intended not just as a review of major technologies for the computer-aided analysis and recognition of medical images (from basic operations to the most advanced classification techniques discussed in subsequent chapters), but also as a presentation of the most up-to-date cognitive techniques for semantically interpreting complex medical patters, namely a broad range of diagnostic images. The authors believe that this original, novel part of the book will not only make an interesting and highly valuable contribution to global research on artificial intelligence methods and computational intelligence algorithms, but will also chart new directions for a biology-inspired branch of modern technologies referred to as cognitive informatics. This interesting, interdisciplinary field of scientific research has recently experienced very rapid development, combining a number of aspects and analyses of perception process modeling and description with natural intelligence features, and then their implementation with the use of advanced computing techniques and new computation methods. In the end, it also uses the systems and models developed (in the form of cognitive systems) to solve complicated problems in the field of pattern analysis, interpretation and semantic categorization. It is through these interesting problems and applications that the reader will be guided in the following chapters. The information presented there may also serve as an introduction to a much longer research process to be developed by broader scientific circles in the coming years as the research on cognitive informatics progresses. The combination of traditional computational informatics with biomedical problems, aspects of philosophy, psychology and linguistics will certainly lead to new, exciting developments which will overcome the current limitations of information technology and fascinate people beyond the realm of academia.

Acknowledgments

The authors wish to thank Dr. Sławomir Bodzioch and Ph.D student Mirosław Trzupek for cooperation in scientific research, and valuable contribution to medical image analysis.

Government support

This work has been supported by the Ministry of Science and Higher Education, Republic of Poland, under scientific research project number N516 025 32/2881.

Marek R. Ogiela and Ryszard Tadeusiewicz

2. Sources of medical images and their general characteristics

2.1. X-ray images

In 1895, the German physicist Wilhelm Roentgen (Fig. 2.1.a) noted that a cathode tube exposes paper coated with a barium compound placed at some distance away. The tube emitted radiation, unknown at that time, which caused the plates to get exposed. Roentgen named that radiation "X rays". His discovery, for which he received the Nobel Prize in 1901 (Fig. 2.1.b and 2.1.c) caused a revolution in medicine, for the first time making it possible to look inside the human body without breaking its integrity, in a way now referred to as noninvasive [2].

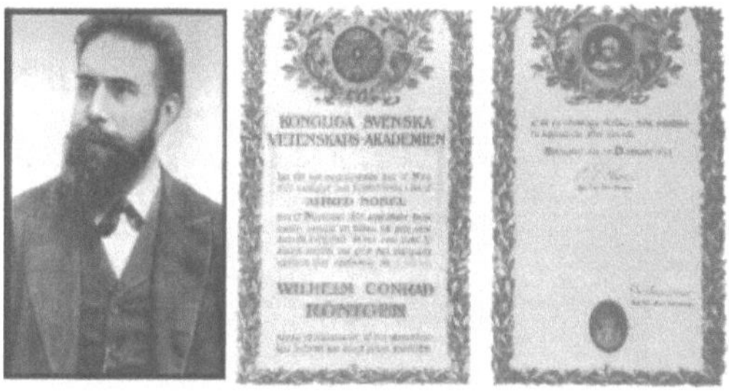

Fig. 2.1. Wilhelm C. Roentgen and a copy of his 1901 Nobel Prize certificate (source Internet)

This technology was subsequently improved by constructors of machines offered to hundreds of radiology practices. The scale of these improvements can be assessed by comparing the historical image from the first ever x-ray examination of a human being (the image of Wilhelm Roentgen's wife's hand – Fig. 2.2.a) with a similar photograph generated by a modern X-ray machine – Fig. 2.2.b.

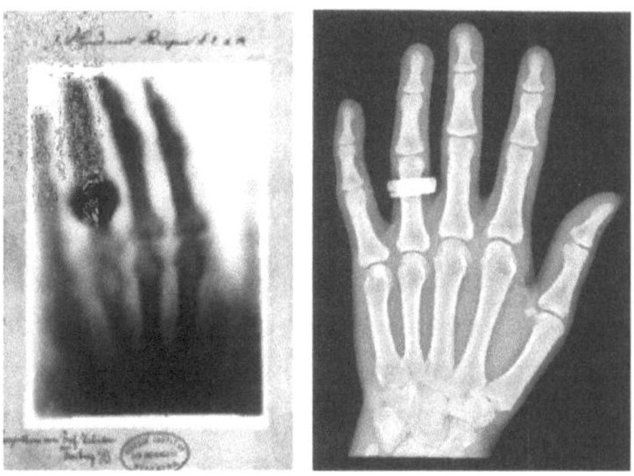

Fig. 2.2. A historic photograph of Roentgen's wife's hand (left) contrasted with a present-day X-ray photograph (right) (source Internet)

M.R. Ogiela and R. Tadeusiewicz: *Sources of medical images and their general characteristics,* Studies in Computational Intelligence (SCI) **84**, 7–45 (2007)
www.springerlink.com

X-ray photography, regardless of its shortcomings (X rays, like any ionizing radiation, are harmful to human health), has become a diagnostic technique widely used until the present. This is why the discussion of various medical imaging techniques presented in this book has to start with X-ray photography, which will occupy the entire first subsection of the second chapter [2].

X-rays are generated in a special tube (Fig. 2.3) in which a beam of electrons accelerated by high voltage hits a metal disk and as a result of the rapid deceleration its kinetic energy is transformed into quanta of emitted X-rays, whose ability to penetrate the human body is the greater the higher the voltage accelerating the electrons in the tube. Electrons hitting the disk make it very hot, so it either has to be cooled on the inside (usually with water) or spun so that electrons hit a new spot while the spot struck previously cools down.

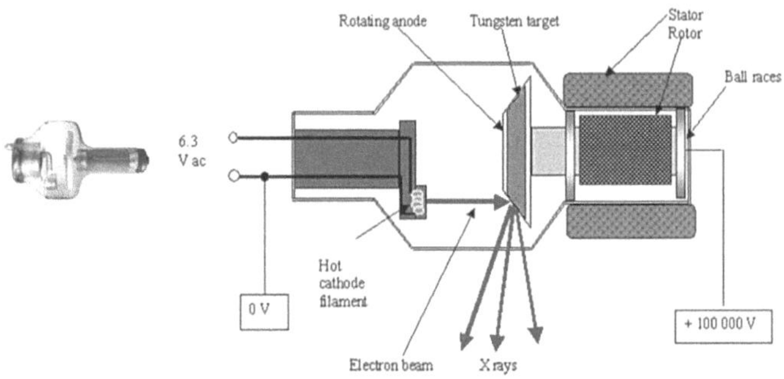

Fig. 2.3. An image and a diagram of an X-ray tube

One feature of X-rays, like of any electromagnetic radiation, is that a certain part of them is weakened after they pass through tissues. This weakening is the result of their interaction with the tissues, and the scale of it depends on the type of tissue they passed through. The intensity of X-ray radiation also depends on the distance and decreases along with the square of the distance. Interactions of X-rays with matter can be divided into three types:

- **The Compton effect** – the electron lying in the trajectory of the beam absorbs some of the energy of the photon forming a part of the beam and changes the direction in which that photon is traveling. As a result, the photon changes its direction and its energy is reduced (Fig. 2.4.a).
- **Rayleigh scattering** – a flexible (i.e. free of energy losses) scattering of photons over atoms which do not absorb energy. Unlike in the Compton effect, the photons of the beam do not lose any energy, only change their direction (Fig. 2.4.b).
- **The photoelectric effect** – a photoelectron is ejected by a photon of the beam. The photon is absorbed by the atom (Fig. 2.4.c).

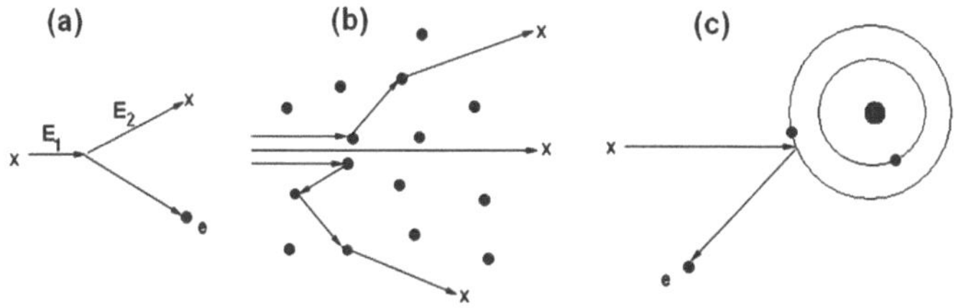

Fig. 2.4. Physical effects that occur when X-rays pass through matter (the patient's body). Described in the text

The main factor causing the weakening of the beam is the Compton effect. The three above effects can be characterized collectively by the following absorption equation (for a uniform medium):

$$I = I_0 e^{-\mu x}$$

where I_0 is the initial intensity of radiation, x is the thickness of the layer through which the beam passes, and μ is the specific absorbance of the substance (its radiodensity). The μ radiodensity depends on the type of substance through which the radiation passes. It is expressed using the Hounsfield scale, presented in Figure 2.5. The reference value (of 0) on that scale is the X-ray absorption by water (which is the main component of all tissues and organs of living organisms). Substances with X-ray absorbance weaker than water (e.g. the air in the lungs) have negative Hounsfield values, down to –1,000 Hounsfield units for light gases. Conversely, substances with X-ray absorbance greater than water (e.g. bones) have positive values, up to +1,000 which is assigned to very hard and dense bones.

X-rays ionize matter and cause luminescence, they also interact with photographic emulsions and semiconductor radiation detectors currently used for X-ray recording and imaging. Unfortunately, these rays also ionize biological tissues, damaging them and potentially leading to many serious diseases. So regardless of the diagnostic benefits accruing from every extra X-ray image, the number of examinations should be limited to the indispensable minimum in order to protect the patient's body from the consequences of exposure to this harmful radiation.

Figure 2.5 shows that tissues of which various organs of the human body are built have μ radiodensities varied enough, so that when X-rays pass through the examined patient's body, depending on the organs and tissues lying along the path from the radiation source to the place of its recording, different levels of energy reach the film coated with the appropriate photosensitive emulsion or the X-ray detector placed on the other side of body. This is the basic effect used in this type of imaging: in the places to which radiation traveled through tissues with a low value on the Hounsfield scale, the film darkens or the CCD detector is excited, while places located behind e.g. parts of the skeleton receive little radiation energy, so light spots are left on the film or electronic detectors return a weak signal (Fig. 2.6).

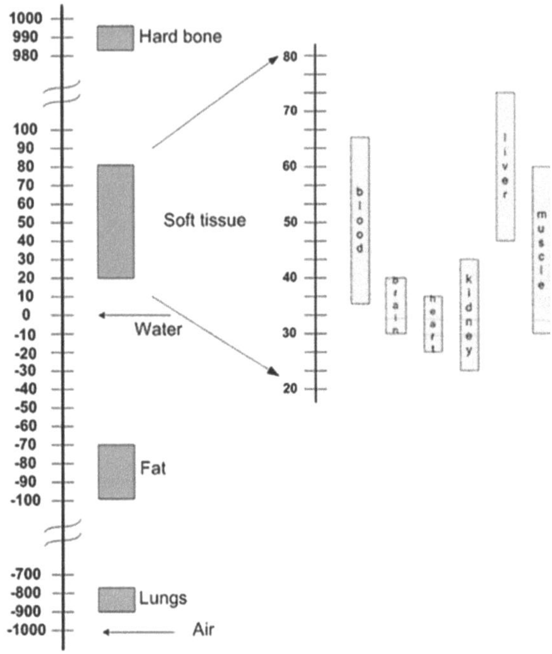

Fig. 2.5. The Hounsfield scale used in x-ray diagnostics

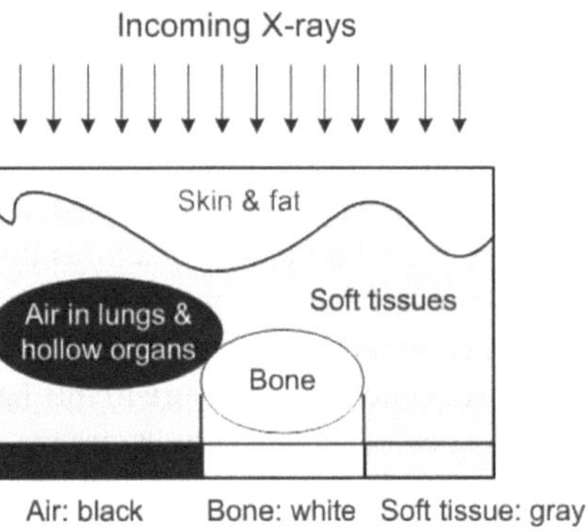

Fig. 2.6. The principle behind the imaging of various tissues in X-ray diagnostics

This suggests that what you see on the acquired medical image are shadows of the organs through which the radiation had to pass, and the more cohesive and dense the organ, the brighter its image (cf. Fig. 2.2.).

It is sometimes said that the X-ray image is the *negative* of the picture of the examined organs, but regardless of the ease with which today's digital radiography could invert grey levels to obtain a positive image, no one does this, as all the traditional methods of interpreting X-ray images used by physicians for years apply to images in the form of negatives.

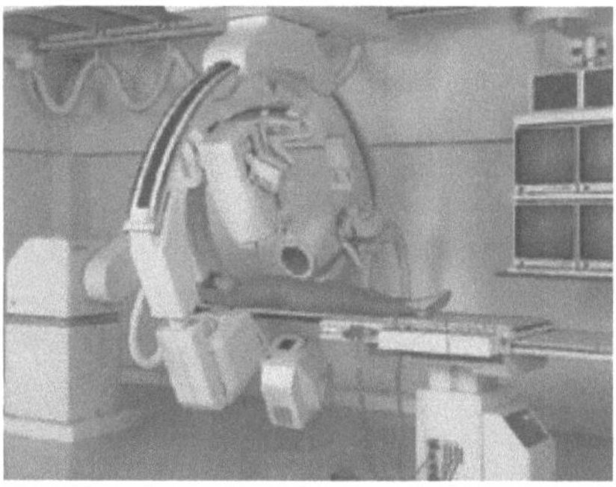

Fig. 2.7. An example of a modern X-ray machine (source Internet)

In practical medical diagnostics, X-ray images are produced by X-ray machines (Fig. 2.7), which may have been improved compared to the historical Roentgen machine, but their operating principle has not changed. They contain at least one X-ray tube, a high voltage generator supplying that tube and devices recording the intensity of radiation after its passage through the patient's body. In less expensive machines, radiation intensity is recorded by a special set of electronic CCD detectors or (in older solutions) on a special photographic plate. Nowadays, the radiation is not recorded directly, but its intensity is measured and then converted into an image. This makes more details visible in the image (Fig. 2.8).

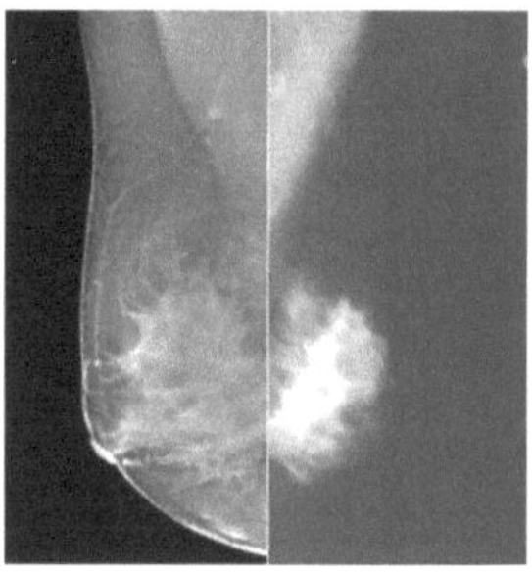

Fig. 2.8. An image produced using modern methods of X-ray intensity measurement and computer-aided imaging (left) compared with an image of the same organ (female breast) recorded on a traditional plate

Contemporary X-ray machines are computer controlled, so examination parameters can be automatically tailored to the patient. They can produce X-ray photographs as well as images for the instant evaluation by doctors. There are also machines for specialized examinations, such as:

- mammography (Fig. 2.9.),
- dental photographs (Fig. 2.10),

- chest and heart diagnostics (Fig. 2.11),
- skeletal system diagnostics (Fig. 2.12).

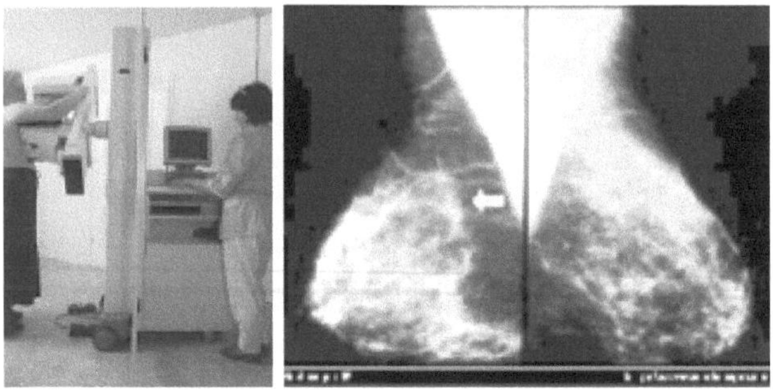

Fig. 2.9. Specialized X-ray examination: mammography (source Internet)

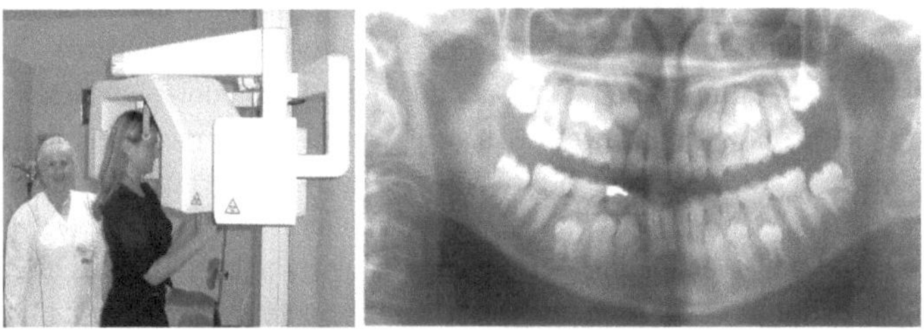

Fig. 2.10. Dental radiography (source Internet)

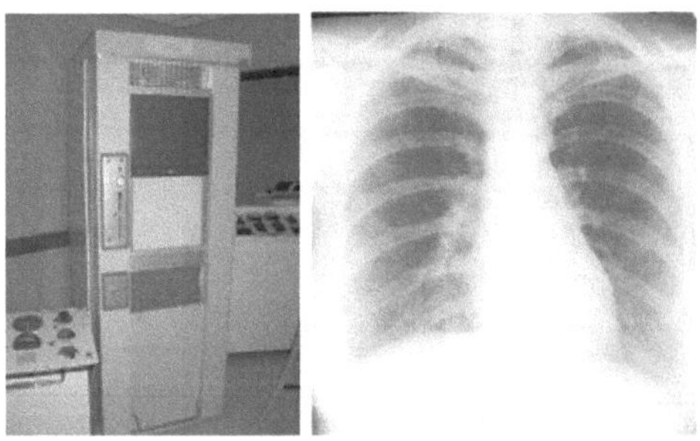

Fig. 2.11. Lung and heart X-ray examinations (source Internet)

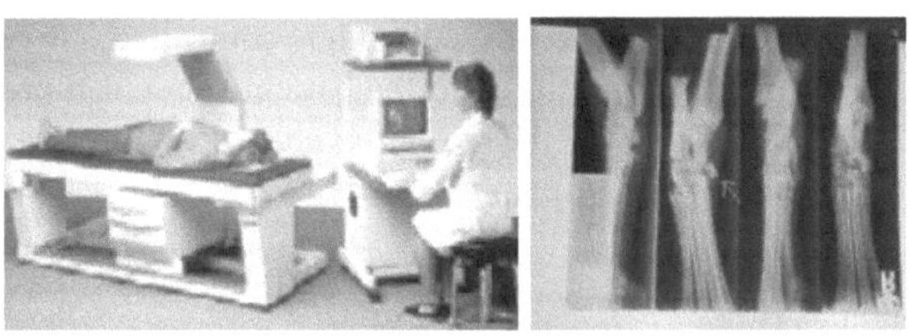

Fig. 2.12. Bone X-ray examination (source Internet)

The radiological image can be recorded and presented in many ways. The following ways of recording these images are used:

- Traditional X-ray photographs obtained using classical photographic plates;
- Digital computer radiology;
- Systems which allow the functions of the organ to be recorded
- CAT scanning (described further down in the chapter).

The improvements in X-ray technology have, however, led to the following problem. Modern detectors can measure the intensity of X-rays so precisely that differences in the radiodensity of single Hounsfield units or even their fractions can be imaged. This means that the digital X-ray image generated in the computer memory consists of pixels represented by between 12 and 16 bits, so the brightness of those points can take one of 4,096 or even 65,536 discrete levels. However, the image is displayed using devices that can only differentiate 256 levels of brightness (or grey levels), while the physician interpreting the image can only differentiate some 60 grey levels with his/her eyesight. This means that due to the limitations of human perception, the proportion of the information that the medical doctor can use to the information obtained by X-ray imaging is like 1:1,000. This is one of the crucial arguments supporting the broad application of computer analysis of medical images to help the physician interpret them, but the problem of the narrow perception range of the human eye also has to be solved somehow.

The problem is most frequently solved by providing a "window" functionality which allows the person to select and see only that fragment of the variability interval of brightnesses expressed on the Hounsfield scale which we believe carries information useful for the diagnostic problem analysed at the time. If we have reasons to believe that the relevant organs and tissues are represented by pixel values from the $[W_1, W_2]$ interval isolated from the complete Hounsfield scale, then we can "cut" that interval using the computer and then rescale it to 256 grey levels. The decision on what W_1, W_2 threshold values to select depends on the physician, as this selection will determine which fragments of the examined body will be captured. It is customary to define W_1, W_2 using the L and W figures, where L is the middle level of the "window", while W is the window width. Examples of the L and W values used in examinations are: window width $W = 300$–600 HU for soft tissues and 800–1600 HU for lungs, window level $L = 0$–30 HU or 30–60 HU for soft tissues and –500–700 HU for lungs. Fig. 2.13 shows what the same X-ray image looks like when different L and W values are chosen.

X-ray images of the same parts of the body may look different depending on how "hard" the radiation generated was. The hardness or penetrating ability of X-rays is adjusted by selecting the voltage accelerating electrons in the tube (cf. Fig. 2.3). As the most frequent examinations made using this technique are skeleton photographs, the most popular voltage is about 70 kV, since at that energy the quanta of X-rays support the best imaging of particular parts of the skeletal system. A similar range of voltages is used to obtain dental images of teeth, while lower voltages of some 50 kV are used to examine the organs in the chest. For soft tissue X-rays (e.g. mammography), a lower interval of voltages is used: 15 kV to 18 kV.

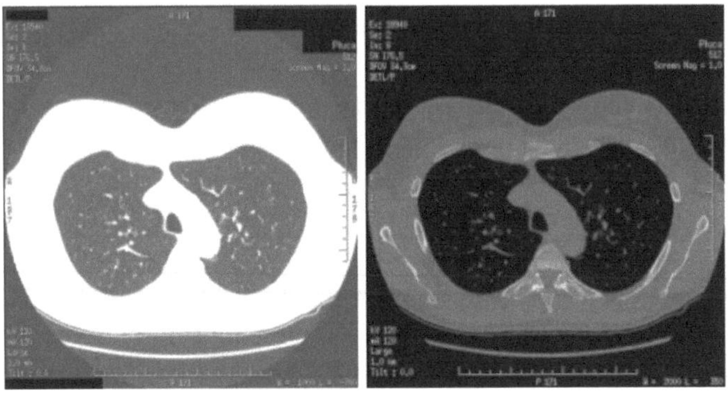

Fig. 2.13. The same X-ray image when different L and W values are chosen: on the left L = –700 HU, W = 1000 HU, on the right L = 350 HU, W = 2000 HU

In some cases, to get the right information about the morphology or the structure of an organ, the patient is given a contrast medium. This medium must have a radiodensity much different from that of the surrounding tissues. It fills the appropriate body cavities (e.g. the inside of the stomach – Fig. 2.14) to give their more precise view.

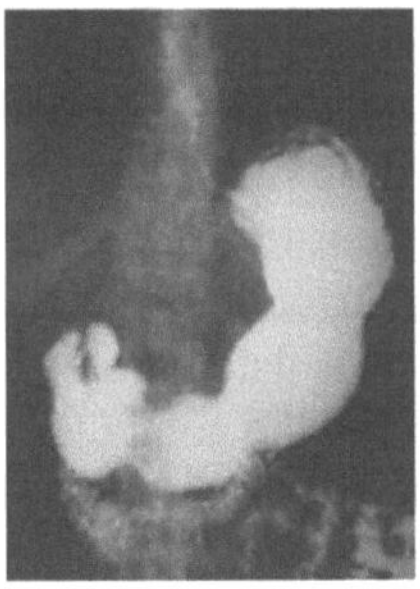

Fig. 2.14. Using a contrast medium for stomach imaging

Imaging the same organ in the same position before and after administering the contrast medium offers interesting opportunities. Subtracting these two images from one another yields an image in which the anatomic details filled with the contrast can be seen (Fig. 2.15). All other anatomic details which did not differ in the two pictures are removed almost completely as a result of the subtraction (*almost* and not completely because you can never get exactly the same position and the same exposure conditions of the organ before and after the contrast was administered). This examination technique is most frequently used to image various vessels (e.g. blood vessels), which is why it is called *angiography*. As this method of discovering anatomic structures is based on the mathematical operation of subtracting, the adjective *subtraction* is added to the name.

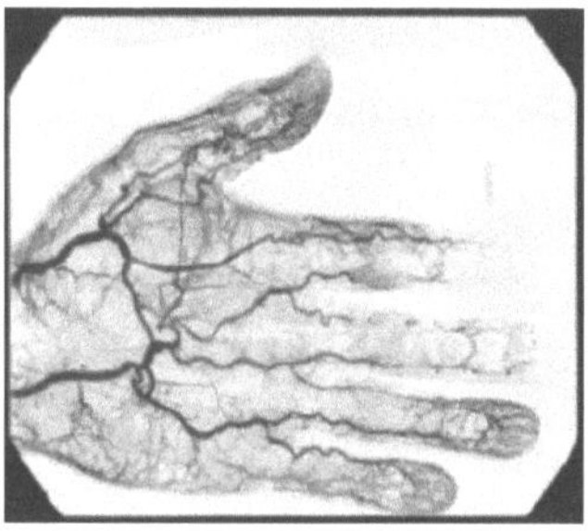

Fig. 2.15. The result of subtraction angiography. Described in the text

2.2. CT images

Apart from magnetic resonance, computed tomography (CT) represents one of the main noninvasive diagnostic techniques used in contemporary medicine. Its popularity is driven both by technological progress yielding subsequent generations of apparatuses with even better parameters of the acquired image, also in the form of 3D reconstructions, and by even faster computers used for the mathematical processing of the measurement data collected [25].

A CT examination consists of probing the patient many times with an appropriately shaped beam of X-rays (Fig. 2.16). When the beam passes through the examined tissues it gets weaker, and its final intensity is measured by the detector. The weakening of the beam (the absorption of radiation) along the path to the detector depends on the type of substance that it penetrates, but for a single probe we get the summary effect of beam weakening by all tissues that it encounters along its path. It is possible to reconstruct the radiation absorption by a specific point on the cross-section of the patient's body as the CT apparatus collects the results of many such images made by beams running in different directions and intersecting many times at different points inside the patient's body. By analyzing the signal recorded by detectors for many such beams, it is possible to calculate the degree of radiation absorption by particular fragments of the examined patient's body, called voxels (Fig. 2.16) through solving the appropriate systems of equations.

On the basis of the results obtained, it is possible to precisely identify the examined tissues and to reconstruct the shapes of organs by making the appropriate calculations. The identification is difficult, as it requires both many measurements and complicated mathematical operations leading to the reconstruction of the spatial structure of the object.

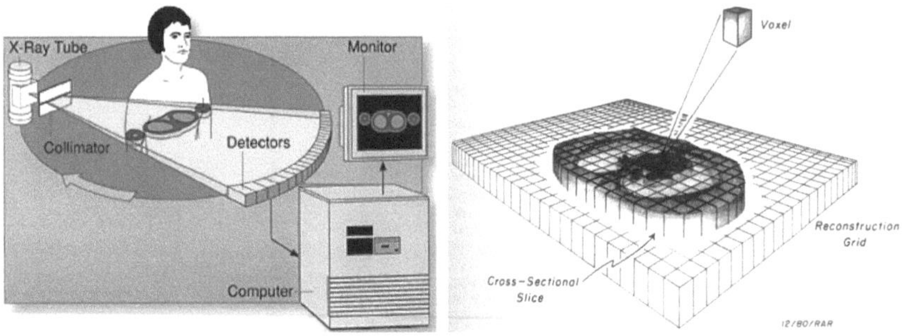

Fig. 2.16. The operating principle of a CT apparatus (source Internet)

The main contribution to the development of CT was made by Godsfrey Hounsfeld (Fig. 2.17), who discovered in 1970 that measurements of the absorption of X-rays allow tissue density to be determined. The technique was first used in 1971, but with only moderate success (see Fig. 2.17).

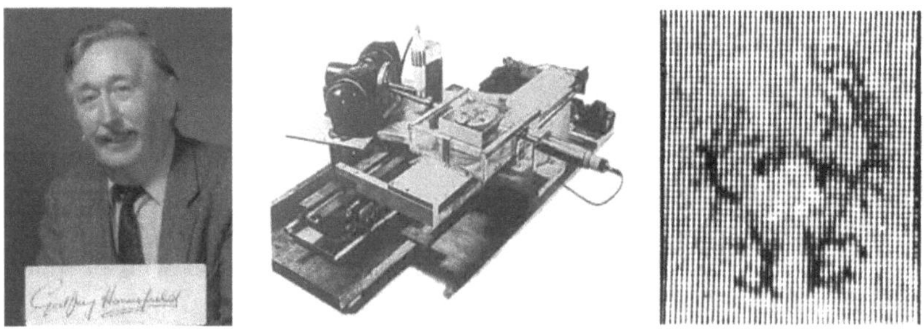

Fig. 2.17. Godfrey Newbold Hounsfield, his CT apparatus and the first CT image (source Internet)

However, the CT technique was gradually improved, mainly as it was not subject to the limitations of traditional X-ray techniques. In a CT image, organs do not obscure one another, so it is possible to make a precise image of the inside of the brain, for example, regardless of the massive shield of the scull behind which it is hidden. In addition, in CT, the density of particular tissues can be calculated so precisely that it is possible to make differentiations absolutely impossible by any other method: for example, congealed blood can be distinguished from flowing, allowing the extent of a stroke to be determined.

Subsequent generations of CT apparatuses could acquire the necessary images within shorter and shorter times while maintaining the principle of a multidirectional probing inside the human body (Fig. 2.18, 2.19).

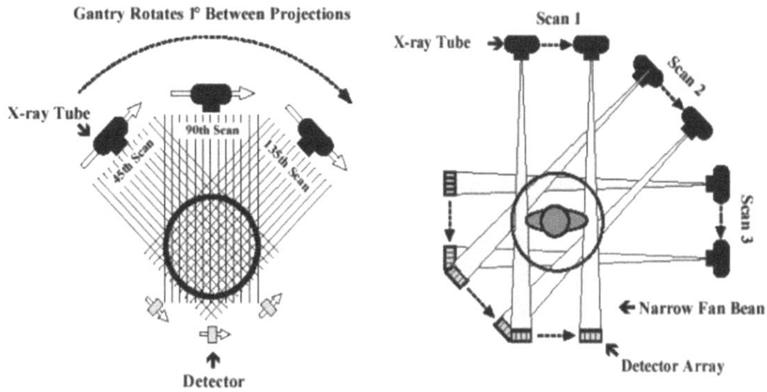

Fig. 2.18. The transition from the first to the second generation of CT apparatuses meant replacing one radiation beam with a whole fan of them and one detector with an array of detectors. This cut the image production time

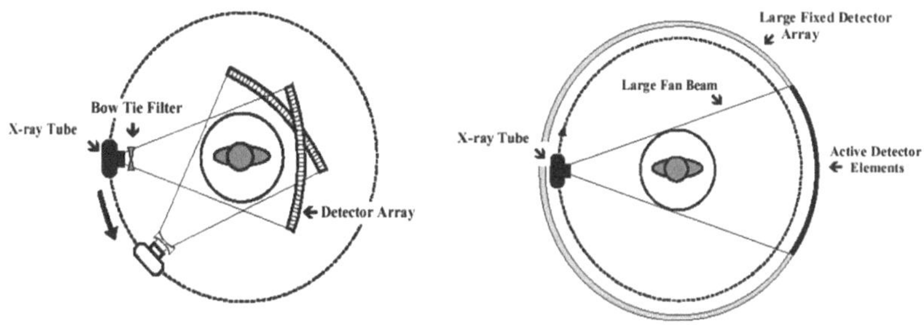

Fig. 2.19. Further progress was achieved mainly by adding more and more detectors, which finally filled the entire ring in the 4th generation CT apparatuses

An innovation in the CT technology was the introduction of a CT apparatus that spun the X-ray tube in a spiral around the patient (Fig. 2.20). The first such examination was made in 1989. The move from the sequential to the spiral technique made it possible to image the human body along any plane. For this reason, spiral computed tomography is now referred to as the volumetric CT or 3D CT. The current CT apparatuses used in medicine allow between one and sixty-four layers to be recorded during one revolution of the tube. This cuts the examination time, reducing the radiation dose.

Computed tomography made it possible to directly assess the brain and other structures inside the skull, which were previously practically out of bounds for radiological examination. In addition, CTs made it possible to determine if these structures had not been shifted. CTs enable the diagnosing specialists to detect many diseases, e.g. tumors and haematomas, which were previously difficult to identify using X-rays. Even though diagnostic capabilities of CT are poorer than those of magnetic resonance, CT is a very popular examination as it is easily available and the acquired images are very legible (Fig. 2.21).

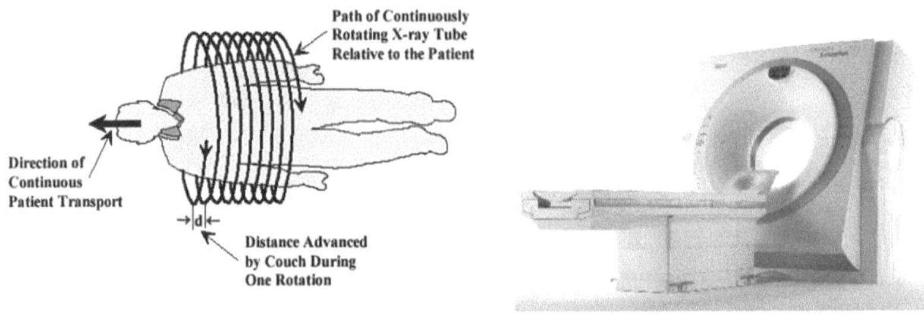

Fig. 2.20. Spiral CT. The operating principle and a view of the apparatus (source Internet)

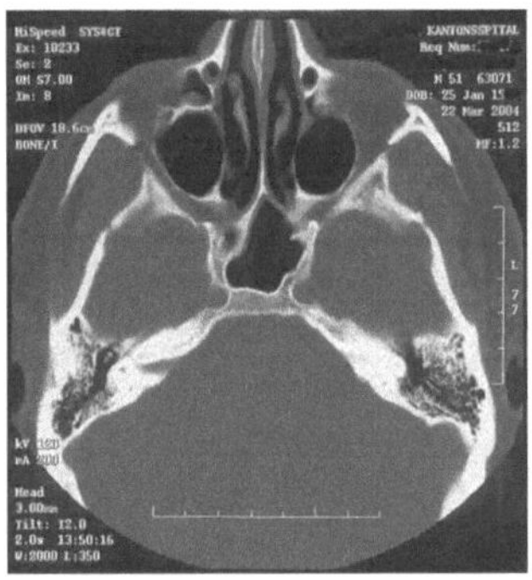

Fig. 2.21. Images produced by CT examinations are of very high quality

The key components of a CT apparatus are shown in Fig. 2.22. The computed tomography apparatus consists of bed on which the examined patient lies, the gantry (a ring-shaped element containing X-ray tubes and radiation detectors) and a computer. Data collected by detectors, including information about the positions of the tube and detectors, is analyzed by the computer to reconstruct the image. In spiral tomography, the bed can move relative to the gantry along its axis of symmetry.

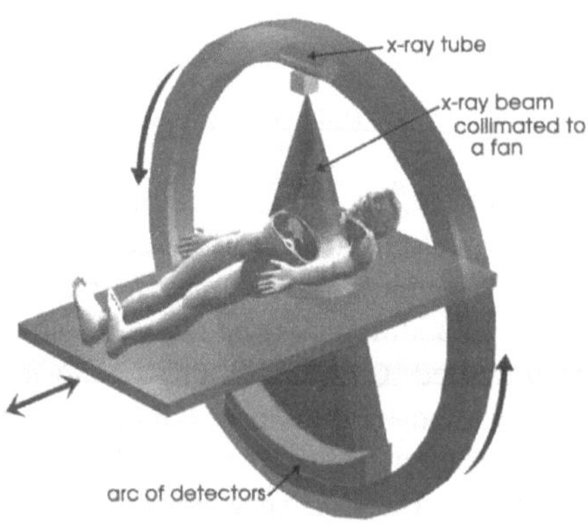

Fig. 2.22. Main structural elements of the CT apparatus (source Internet)

The part of the patient's body to be scanned is divided into layers (Fig. 2.23), every one of which consists of volume elements called voxels (volumetric pixels) (see Fig. 2.16). Cross-sections may lie in three planes (Fig. 2.24).

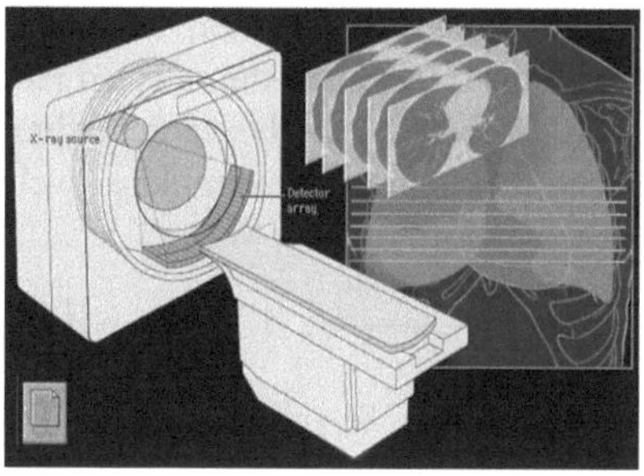

Fig. 2.23. A CT examination produces a series of images representing subsequent cross-sections of the examined fragment of the patient's body (source Internet)

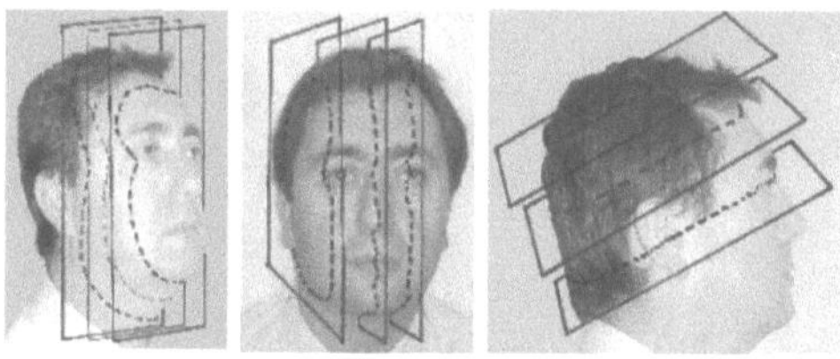

Fig. 2.24. The CT apparatus can produce images of body cross-sections along different planes (source Internet)

A single cross-section, 0.75 mm – 10 mm thick, is a matrix of voxels subsequently represented by pixels of the produced image. The matrix size for images used in this publication is 512 × 512 voxels (pixels). The resolution of a voxel is about 0.5 × 0.5 × 0.6 mm. In general, reducing the volume of a voxel improves image quality, but brings about an increase in the radiation dose.

Series of cross-sections obtained by a CT examination can be analyzed as sequences of images on the basis of which the physician formulates the diagnosis and prescribes the treatment, but a more attractive functionality is offered by the ability of the computer to reconstruct a spatial image of the organ analyzed (Fig. 2.25).

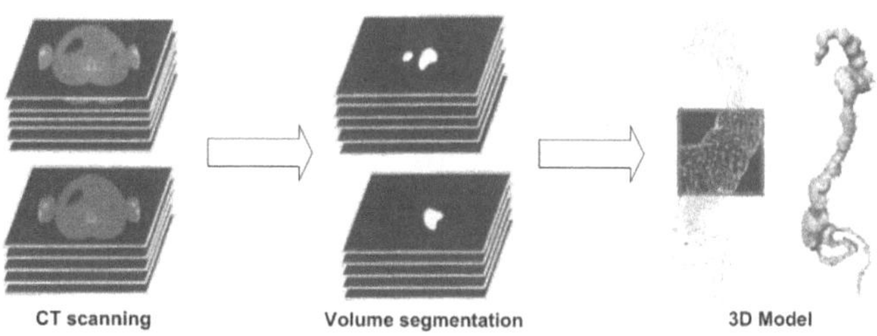

Fig. 2.25. The principle for creating a three-dimensional model based on a series of cross-sections from a CT scan

Tissue densities calculated by the CT apparatus are expressed on the Hounsfield scale discussed in the previous subsection (as part of the discussion of X-ray image characteristics). For the human body, these values range from –1000 HU to 1000 HU and cannot be precisely shown to a person who would like to assess these images visually. This is why for CT images, the selected Hounsfield values range is also replaced with the set (0, 1, ..., 255). In this examination, it is also customary to define the W_1, W_2 limits and then represent the middle level of the interval with the L value and the width of the window with the W:

$$L = \frac{W_1 + W_2}{2}, \; W = W_2 - W_1.$$

The right selection of the L and W values used in the examination not only determines what is visible in the image (Fig. 2.26) but also makes it possible to control the subjective impression received by the physician analyzing the image (Fig. 2.27).

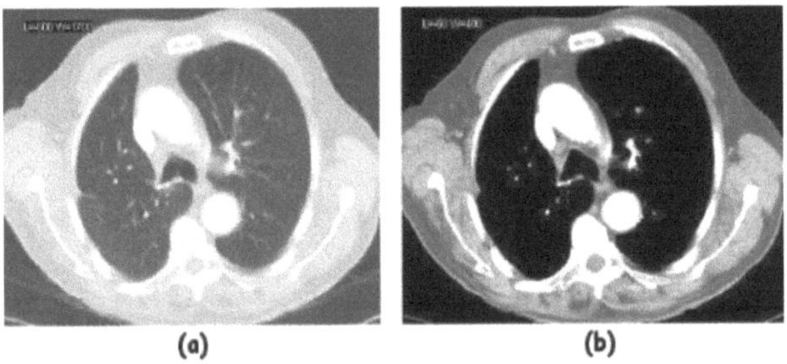

Fig. 2.26. Image (a) obtained for L = –600, W = 1700 shows much more details, while in image (b) produced at L = 50, W = 400 many items are not visible, but it is easier to focus on the distinguished objects

CT images showing the same anatomical structures of different patients can be compared more easily by applying a grid which shows individual deformations to be applied to the image of the examined patient to enable his/her comparison with the reference image. This technique is discussed in one of the subsequent chapters.

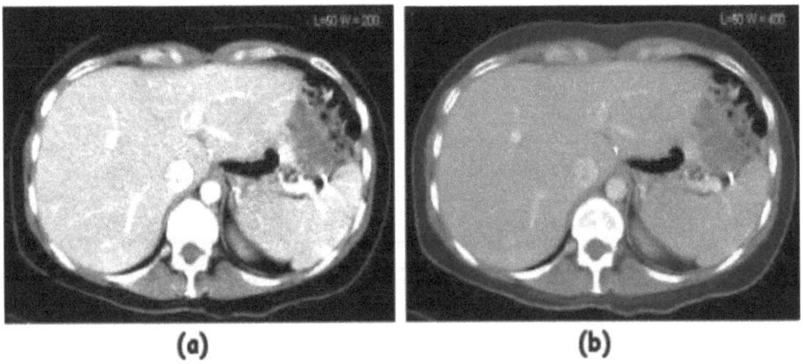

Fig. 2.27. Using a wider window reduces the contrast of the image, so it appears less noisy (image (a) L = 50 and W = 200, image (b) at L = 50 and W = 400)

2.3. NMR images

One of the newest and best methods of diagnostic imaging is the magnetic resonance (MR) technique, which uses the phenomenon of nuclear magnetic resonance (NMR) [17]. Since the word "nuclear" is tainted by unpleasant associations with atom bombs, Chernobyl and radioactivity, this method is sometimes also called Magnetic Resonance Imaging (MRI). However, MRI methods us atomic nuclei, and more precisely the fact that some of them have a spin, so they exhibit a magnetic moment (Fig. 2.28). This technique was first used for clinical examinations in 1982.

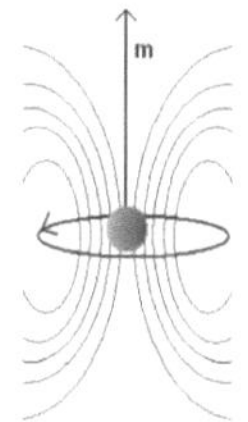

Fig. 2.28. NMR imaging makes use of the spin of certain atomic nuclei, which gives them a natural magnetic moment

Magnetic resonance mainly uses hydrogen analysis, which means that the generation of electromagnetic radiation by hydrogen atom nuclei (protons) in the organism is analysed. This is because these nuclei return a very clear signal when they are properly magnetically excited and because hydrogen is widely present in the human body, for instance in the water which constitutes one of the main building blocks of our organisms.

Another element whose nuclei exhibit a non-zero spin, and can therefore be used for nuclear magnetic resonance imaging, is phosphorus. The signal obtained from phosphorus nuclei is more difficult to receive and interpret, but phosphorus plays a key role in the activity of live tissues and whole organs. Phosphorus atoms are present in molecules of one important chemical compound: Adenosine 5'-triphosphate (ATP – Fig. 2.29). This substance is the main source of energy for all biological processes, so by using NMR to find out where ATP molecules are situated in the examined organ we can also discover which parts of the organ are active, and which are less active. This is of major importance for attempts to link medical images not just to the morphology of specific organs, but also to their function.

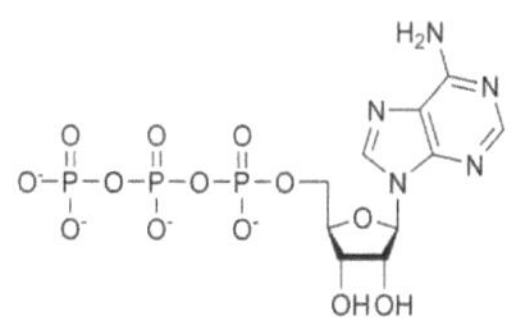

Fig. 2.29. ATP is a chemical compound whose location can be determined using the NMR

Magnetic resonance is a method for visualizing internal organs of a human (or another biological) being in which the image is constructed in the computer as a result of acquiring and recording a physical signal (an electromagnetic wave of a radio frequency) generated by the organ itself. Consequently, this imaging technique is dramatically different from the previously discussed X-ray examinations (traditional or tomography), in which the source of the signal is an external tube emitting X-rays. In X-ray examinations, the organs are "lit up" with external radiation, and then you view their shadows. In NMR, the organs "shine" themselves, the source of that radiation being the atomic nuclei of elements making up the molecules of which organs are built.

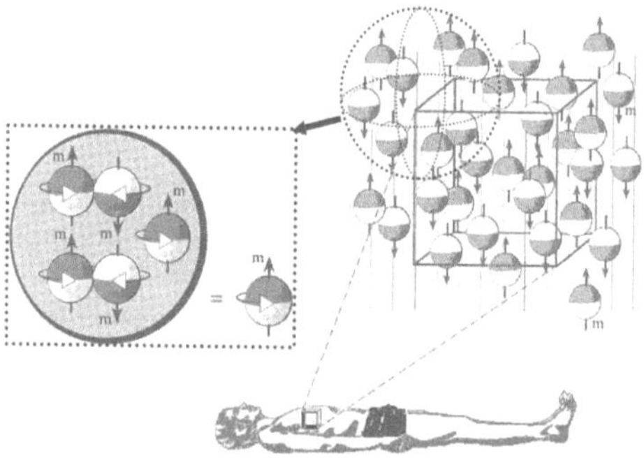

Fig. 2.30. An external magnetic field aligns nuclear spins inside the patient's body (source Internet)

For these natural atoms to start "shining", they have to be appropriately excited. NMR uses a strong magnetic field for imaging. This field causes the nuclei of atoms in the patient's body to be aligned and spatially oriented (Fig. 2.30), so when an external impulse comes to excite them, they respond with a "harmonious tune", giving a clear and easily recordable signal revealing where they are more abundant, and where less. MR apparatuses use permanent, superconducting and resistance magnets to generate that aligning magnetic field. These magnets differ in the structure and intensity of the field they emit. The magnetic field intensity determines diagnostic capabilities of the MR apparatus: for spectroscopy, quick vascular examinations or functional examinations you need an apparatus with a high field intensity. In medicine, MR apparatuses with the magnetic field intensities ranging from 0.1 to 3.0 Tesla are used.

The key element of the magnetic resonance tomograph (Fig. 2.31) is the chamber in which the examined patient lies [17]. The chamber is inside the main magnet generating the external (to the patient's body) magnetic field B_0 to align the magnetic moments of hydrogen (and phosphorus, as mentioned above) atoms. These aligned magnetic moments of nuclei of all atoms make up the M magnetization vector generated by the entire examined sample. In order to make it uniform, correcting coils which induce an additional magnetic field compensating the non-uniformities of the B_0 field are used. The effect of the linear field change (gradient), fundamental for NMR examinations, is obtained by using additional gradient coils. On top of this, you need coils which force the "hits" of the external magnetic field, causing the atomic nuclei to resonate, as described above. The device which acquires the signal from the resonating atomic nuclei is the receiving coil with an axis perpendicular to that of the main magnet. This function is frequently provided by the same coils which are used to cause the impulse exciting the resonance. A schematic diagram of the above elements is presented in Figure 2.32.

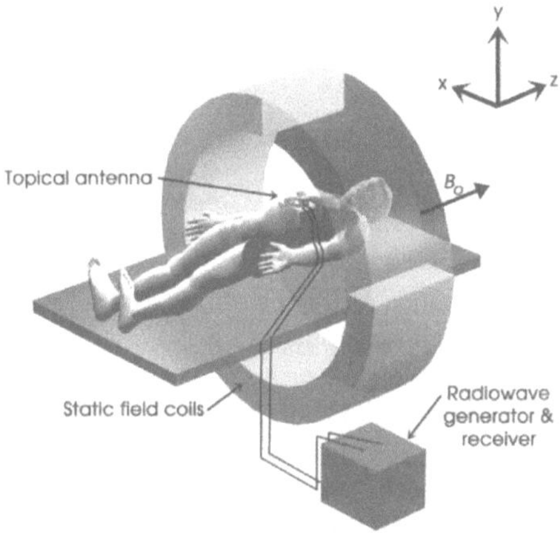

Fig. 2.31. A simplified diagram of an NMR apparatus (source Internet)

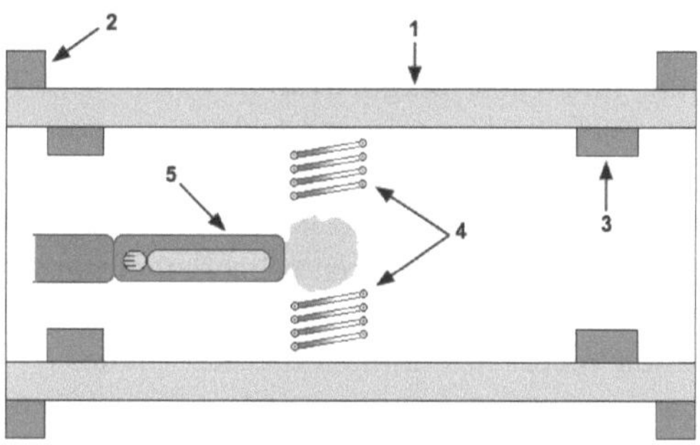

Fig. 2.32. The schematic distribution of particular elements in an NMR apparatus: 1 – main magnet, 2 – correcting coils, 3 – gradient coils, 4 – forcing and receiving coils, 5 – examined patient

The principle of acquiring the signal used for MRI imaging can be summarized as follows. The tissue located in the external B_0 field, which has a specific, defined magnetization M, is exposed to an electromagnetic impulse of a specific, defined frequency (the ω_0 Larmor frequency) whose direction is perpendicular to the direction of M and B_0. In those conditions, a nuclear resonance occurs. It consists in energy absorption by atomic nuclei whose magnetic moments contributed to the M magnetization. As a result of this phenomenon, the M vector transits to the plane perpendicular to B_0 (the transverse plane) on which it makes rotary (precession) movements at the Larmor frequency (Fig. 2.33). Please note that the relationship between the ω_0 Larmor frequency and the type of nucleus means that an impulse of the right frequency will excite only one type of nuclei.

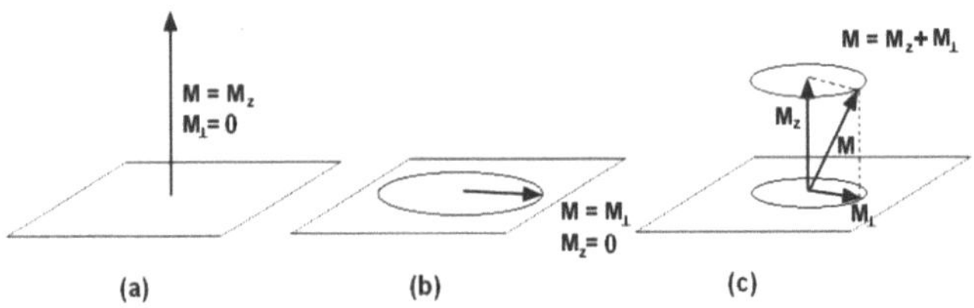

Fig. 2.33. Situation of the magnetization vector of the tissue examined: (a) before exciting, (b) at the moment of excitation, (c) during the relaxation process after the excitation.

An important phenomenon occurs at the level of single atomic nuclei. All the **m** magnetic moments of individual nuclei which make up the M magnetization spin after the excitation, in the transverse plane, at the same frequency (Larmor frequency) and in consistent phases.

The magnetization vector can be split into the sum of two components:

$$\mathbf{M} = \mathbf{M}_\perp + \mathbf{M}_z,$$

where $\mathbf{M}_\perp$ is the transverse magnetization component lying in the plane perpendicular to the B_0 field direction, while $\mathbf{M}_z$ is the longitudinal component parallel to the B_0 direction. Initially (before the excitation), there is no perpendicular component, so $M_\perp = 0$, as transverse components of magnetic moments of individual nuclei are randomly oriented and therefore neutralize one another. On the other hand, in the moment directly after the excitation, $\mathbf{M}_z = 0$ and the magnetization vector lies in the transverse plane.

If the appropriately oriented receiving coil is placed in the vicinity of such an excited tissue, then in accordance with the Faraday's law of electromagnetic induction, alternating current with the frequency of ω_0 will appear in the coil. This is called the free induction decay (FID) signal. The magnitude of this current depends on the value of the magnetization M, and more precisely on the value of its transverse component $M_\perp$, which at the initial moment satfies the equation $M = M_\perp$. The current induced as a result of the magnetic resonance effect constitutes a signal, the knowledge of which allows an image of the examined tissue to be created.

After the impulse which caused the resonance ends, a phenomenon referred to as *the relaxation* occurs (see Fig. 2.33).

Relaxation consists of two independent processes:

1. The $\mathbf{M_z}$ longitudinal component of magnetization is restored. This is due to the constant presence of the $\mathbf{B_0}$ external magnetic field.
2. The $\mathbf{M}_\perp$ transverse component decays to zero. The disappearance of $\mathbf{M}_\perp$ is brought about by two reasons. The first is the non-uniformity of the $\mathbf{B_0}$ magnetic field, the second comes from interactions between the **m** magnetic moments of adjacent nuclei.

The return of the $\mathbf{M_z}$ magnetization to its original value and the total decay of the $\mathbf{M}_\perp$ value take place within different time scales, characterized by two time-constants T_1 and T_2, respectively referred to as the time of longitudinal relaxation and the time of transverse relaxation (Fig. 2.34). The T_1 parameter is defined as the time needed for $\mathbf{M_z}$ to fall to 63% of its initial value (i.e. before the excitation), while T_2 is the time after which 63% of the $\mathbf{M}_\perp$ transverse magnetization following the excitation decays.

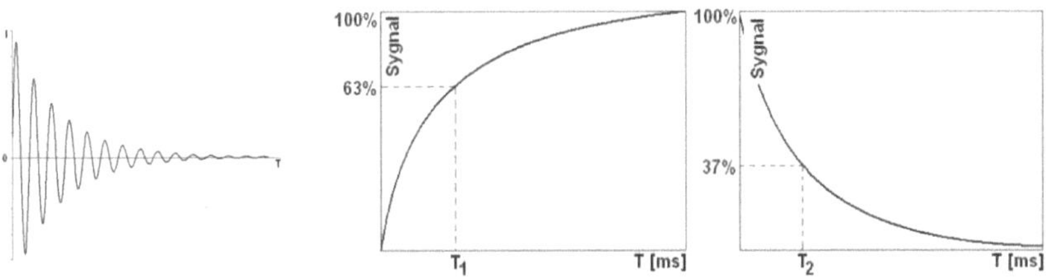

Fig. 2.34. The decay of the transverse magnetization resonance signal during the relaxation (left) and definitions of T_1 and T_2 time-constants (right)

The T_1 and T_2 times range from 0.08 s to 2.5 s for human tissues, depending on the tissue type. The extreme cases are represented by fatty tissue, with short relaxation times, and water, for which T_1 and T_2 are very long. So, for example, T_2 of water is 0.2 s, and T_2 of fat is 0.08 s.

Magnetic resonance diagnostics makes use of not single stimulating impulses, but their sequences. What is important are two time parameters, namely the Time of Repetition (TR) and the Time of Echo (TE), both measured in milliseconds. TR is the time between two subsequent impulses, while TE between the impulse and the maximum signal (current) in the coil (Fig. 2.35).

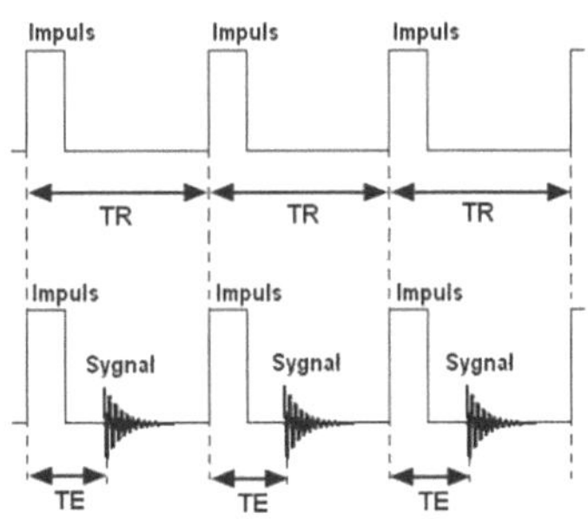

Fig. 2.35. Definitions of TR and TE

TR and TE are apparatus settings, so they can be changed by the operator of the MR scanner. Their right values secure the desired contrast of images obtained from the examination.

Magnetic resonance scanners can be used with three methods of contrasting tissues. The first two use the differences in relaxation times, T_1 or T_2, between different substances of which the human body is made. The third is based on differences in proton densities (PD) of those substances.

For **T1 weighted images** (also called T1 imaging), the important thing is the difference between the rate at which a different tissues recover their $\mathbf{M_z}$ longitudinal magnetization component. As the T_1 time of fat is shorter than the T_1 of water, after the expiry of TR, the value of the longitudinal component of the magnetization vector of fat is greater than of water. As a result, when both magnetization vectors are again "laid" in the transverse plane following the next impulse, the **M** magnetization length for fat is longer, the impulse in the coil stronger, and thus the image of this tissue brighter. In this case, the setting that makes it possible to manipulate the contrast is the time of repetition – TR - which determines to what extent $\mathbf{M_z}$ components are recovered. In order to obtain satisfactory imaging, short TR and TE are used.

To produce **T2 weighted images** (T2 imaging, T2 contrasting), the difference in the speed with which the transverse component of magnetization dissipates in various tissues is used. Just as in the previous case, the T_2 transverse relaxation time of fat is shorter than that of water. So if we wait the appropriate TE time after the exciting impulse, we get a relatively strong signal from where water is present and a weak signal (or none at all) from fatty tissue. Consequently, in T2 imaging, unlike in T1, fatty tissues are dark while water is bright. The setting influencing the contrast quality is the TE echo time. It is easy to observe that if too short a TE is selected, even the transverse component with a short T_2 (which quickly dissipates) will not manage to dissipate sufficiently to make a clearly visible difference between the signal it generates and signals generated by transverse components of other tissues. For T2 weighted images, a good contrast is obtained if the TR and TE times are long.

The third type of contrasting is the proton density weighing (PD). This is based on differences in the density of protons (hydrogen atomic nuclei) in different tissues and disregards the differences in relaxation times of particular tissue types. In order to fulfill the last condition, you set a long TR repetition time and a short TE echo time. The long TR allows the $\mathbf{M_z}$ longitudinal components of both fat and areas dominated by water (taking those two extreme examples) to recover before another stimulating impulse is emitted. This mitigates the effect described above which is used for T1 imaging. Setting a short TE time after which the signal is read guarantees that the dissipation of $\mathbf{M_\perp}$ transverse magnetization components of various tissues will be practically the same. If so, then the only factor determining the signal strength ($\mathbf{M_\perp}$ length) is quantity of protons whose **m** magnetic moments contribute to **M,** which is proportional to the density. The more protons in a given tissue, the greater its **M** magnetization, the stronger the signal and the brighter the image.

Figure 2.36 shows example images of brain structures made using T1, T2 and PD contrasting.

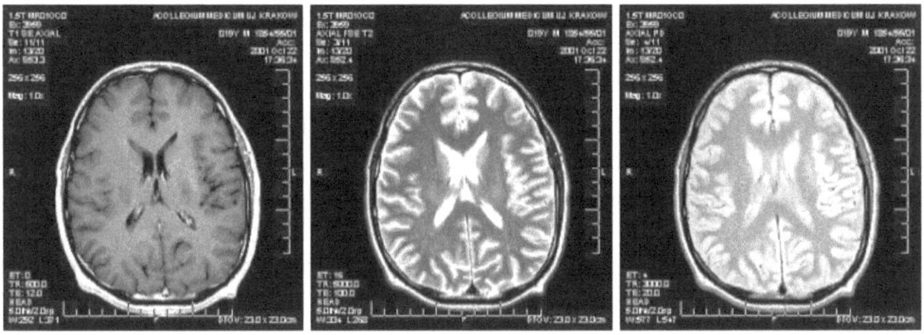

Fig. 2.36. The same brain image made with different contrasts (from the left) T1, T2 and PD

Magnetic resonance is used particularly in the clinical diagnostics of the central nervous system, but examinations of the head and spine are also made. An MR examination of the head allows the brain tissue to be assessed, as the white matter and the grey matter (cerebral cortex), deep structures, the ventricle system, and intracranial sections of cranial nerves can be distinguished. Since there are no bone artifacts typical for the computed tomography of the head, an MR examination is the main method for assessing the structures of the posterior cranial cavity, with particular emphasis on the pons and the medulla (Fig. 2.37).

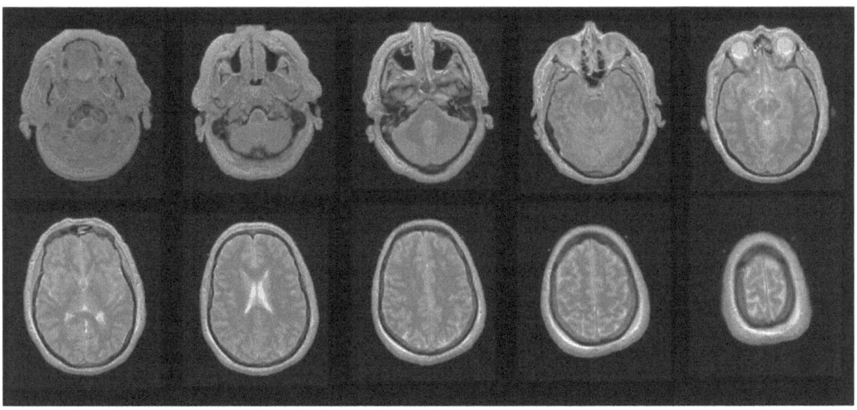

Fig. 2.37. An example NMR image of the brain

A magnetic resonance examination also makes it possible to distinguish all the main elements of the spine, including vertebral bodies and arches as well as the contents of the spinal canal. Magnetic resonance is the only method allowing the spinal cord to be directly imaged. It is worth noting that the NMR technique also allows the image of the blood flowing through arteries and veins to be visualised. Some methods of imaging require no contrast media to be administered. Such solutions are used to examine cartoid arteries upstream of the brain and to assess intracranial arteries or veins.

Magnetic resonance is also used for examining joints, both large ones like knees, shoulders, hips or ankles, and small one like those in the wrist, palm and instep.

During the early clinical applications of magnetic resonance, it was difficult to assess of organs in the abdominal cavity due to the presence of mobile artifacts, for example caused by breathing or peristaltic movements of the intestines. The modern, fast MR apparatuses that allow examinations to be made on a held breath or feature a breath gating function for longer sequences have significantly reduced breathing-related distortions of the image. Consequently, organs from the abdominal cavity, including the liver, pancreas, spleen and kidneys, can now be assessed using magnetic resonance.

Two-dimensional MR images are usually 256 × 256 pixels in size or larger, whereas the depth of brightness is defined with 16 bits. If a CT and an NMR image of the same organ (Fig. 2.38) are compared, the CT scan shows more anatomical details, while the NMR image differentiates tissues of different biological functions better.

The primary advantage of NMR images is that in these images, healthy tissue can easily be told apart from diseased areas. For example, Figure 2.38 shows the NMR image of a cyst in the brain (on the left), and on the right side of the same image, a brain tumor area can easily be seen. Even a poorly experienced observer can see signs of pathology in these images. To compare, it is worth looking at Figure 2.37, which will help less experienced readers to see what the corresponding image without disease symptoms looks like.

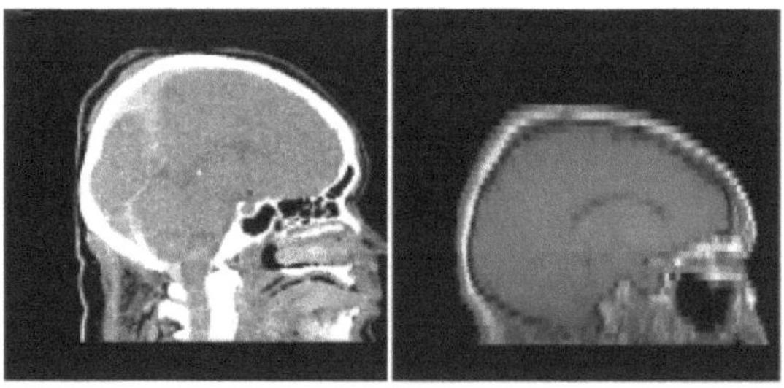

Fig. 2.38. Comparing a CT (left) and NMR (right)

When there is a good technique for imaging the anatomy of an organ (computed tomography) and there are also separate, good methods for imaging this organ clearly distinguishing functional and disfunctional features of tissues, it seems obvious and natural to combine these two images so as to get an image presenting both complete morphological information (from the CT) and information on the detected pathology (from the NMR e.g Fig 2.39).

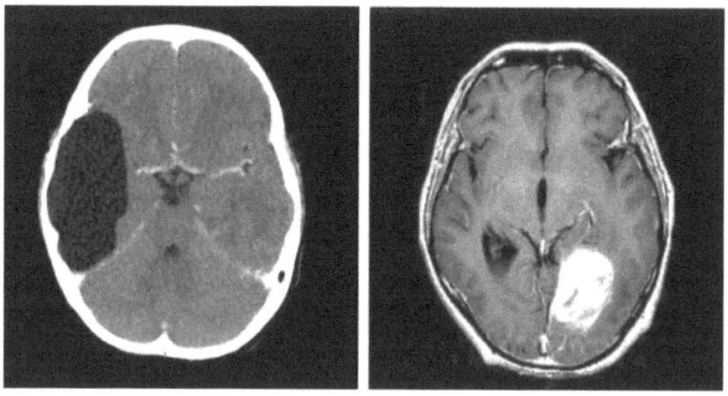

Fig. 2.39. Brain pathologies detected by NMR examinations

This idea is possible, but unfortunately difficult to put into practice. The opportunities for and methods of creating such hybrid images will be discussed in one of the subsequent chapters.

2.4. Nuclear imaging

The NMR technique described above was based on the fact that the appropriate manipulation of the magnetic field caused nuclei of atoms making up the examined tissues and organs to emit a signal. Radionuclide imaging techniques which we are going to discuss now use the fact that nuclei of isotopes of biologically active elements spontaneously emit radiation which can be recorded by modern apparatuses. The intensity of the radiation is recorded continuously together with the location from which the radiation comes (i.e. indicating the fragment of the organ in which the isotope accumulated). This allows you to follow the presence of the radionuclide, changing over time, in specific locations of the body, the route it takes to reach particular organs, the method of its excretion and the like. We should add, even if this is generally known, that a radioactive isotope undergoes chemical reactions exactly like its non-radioactive, biologically-active equivalent. So if an organ absorbs, accumulates or excretes a given chemical compound, it will do so also if the compound contains a radionuclide. However, an isotope-labeled compound can be located using apparatuses external to the patient's body, even in trace amounts. What is more, the apparatus can follow the quantity of the isotope-labeled substance in different parts of the body on a current basis. All these observations give physicians valuable information, completely inaccessible by any other means.

The key to using the above method is the availability of isotope-labeled, biologically active substances produced by pharmaceutical companies which specialize in such operations. Examples of radionuclides used in medicine with the organs for whose examination they can be used are presented in the tables in Fig. 2.40.

MEDICAL RADIONUCLIDES	APPLICATIONS
• Germanium - 68	• PET Calibration Source
• Paladium - 103	• Prostate Cancer Treatment
• Iodine - 125	• Prostate Cancer Treatment
• Ge - 68/Ga - 68 G Generator	• PET Imaging & Research
NUCLEAR MEDICINE	**APPLICATIONS**
• Molybdenum - 99	• Mo99/Tc99 Imaging
• Strontium - 82	• Positron Emission Tomography (PET)
• Iodine - 131	• Thyroid Cancer & Hypertension Treatment
NEW DEVELOPMENTS	**APPLICATIONS**
• Strontium - 89	• Bone Cancer Pain Palliation
• Tin - 117	• Bone Cancer Pain Palliation PET Calibration Source

Fig. 2.40. Examples of radioactive isotopes used in nuclear medicine (source Internet)

It is worth calming a concern frequent among both patients and physicians by saying that radionuclides used in nuclear medicine, if properly selected and carefully examined for their radioactivity level, constitute practically no threat to the health and life of both patients and the personnel. From the patient's point of view, the dose of ionizing radiation he/she receives during a properly conducted isotope examination is lower than the dose to which his/her body is exposed during a typical X-ray.

Medical staff who come into contact with isotopes again and again (unlike the patient, who is usually exposed to them only once), must exercise some caution as even small doses of radiation can accumulate in the body. However, if the appropriate procedures are followed, there is no health hazard.

The procedure of an examination with the use of radionuclides may differ depending on the organ to be examined. For some, it is enough to drink the isotope-containing pharmaceutical in the form of a solution, other such pharmaceuticals are gaseous and can be breathed in, however the most commonplace is an intravenously injected pharmaceutical. After the pharmaceutical is administered, the patient is placed in the field of view of a gamma camera, which follows and records the path taken by the isotope in the body, and in particular the locations where it is accumulated (Fig. 2.41).

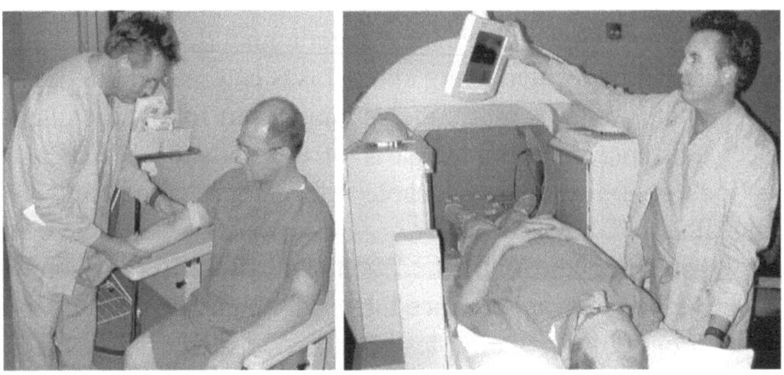

Fig. 2.41. Radionuclide examination. Radioactive pharmaceutical administration on the left, tracing its path in the patient's body on the right (source Internet)

As this book discusses mainly the techniques for medical imaging and computer processing of images, we will focus on apparatuses recording images and the properties of those images, while the physics of isotopes and the design of radiation detectors will be omitted.

The operating principle of the technique for radionuclide imaging can easily be discussed by referring to the diagram of the apparatus used by the pioneer of this examination method, **Ben Classen,** in 1950 (Fig. 2.42).

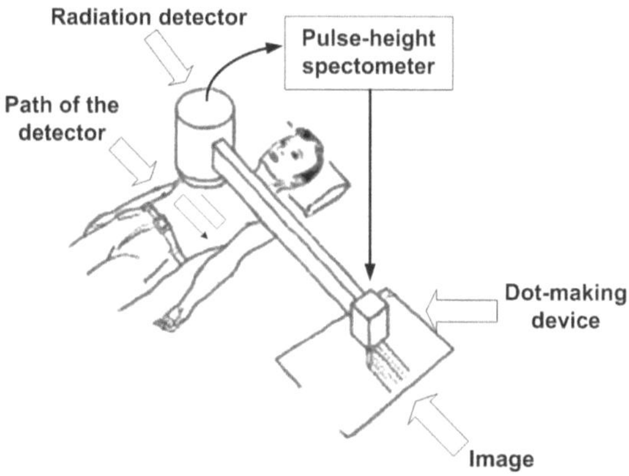

Fig. 2.42. The historical (currently abandoned) method of imaging radionuclide distribution in the human body

In the above examination method, after administering the radionuclide to the patient, a radiation detector was moved above his/her body and places where the detector measured higher radiation were marked on paper. The resultant paper map showed where there was a lot of the radionuclide, and where little. Nowadays, the same purpose is achieved easier, faster and more effectively with devices called gamma cameras (Fig. 2.43).

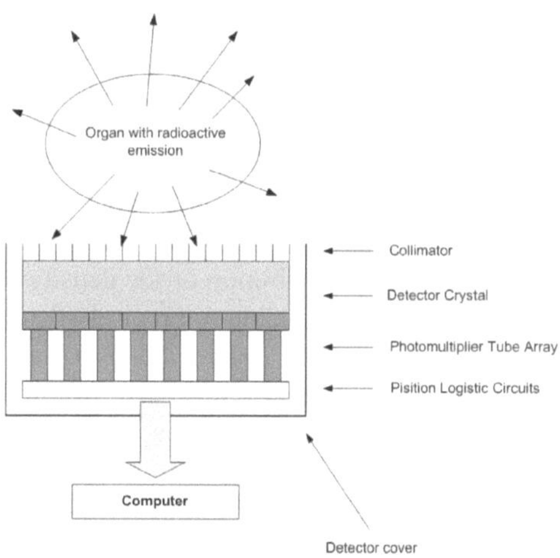

Fig. 2.43. A simplified design diagram of a gamma camera

These devices, which make use of many independent detectors (frequently equipped with photomultipliers to raise their sensitivity), can receive the radiation emitted by radioactive isotopes in tissues and organs from many points at the same time. This is illustrated (schematically and at a great simplification) in Figure 2.44, which also shows some other elements incorporated in the set of apparatuses designed for this type of examinations.

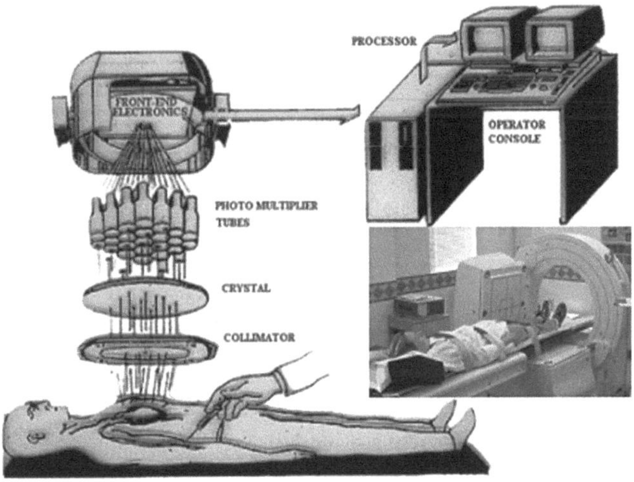

Fig. 2.44. The diagram and the appearance of a typical apparatus set for radionuclide image diagnostics (source Internet)

It is worth noting that a gamma camera, which receives very weak radiation from inside the patient's body, must be shielded very well from radiation from other sources, of which there are very many all around us. This is why the gamma camera is armored with a thick screen usually made of lead, which makes it very heavy and requires very strong equipment to transport it over the patient's body. This is obvious from the color insert in Fig. 2.44, which shows the complete example of an apparatus of the type discussed here.

Regardless of the huge weight of the gamma camera, diagnostic devices capable of receiving images from many different directions are now available: Fig. 2.45. This helps in formulating conclusions on the activity of particular parts of human organs assessed based on the distribution of the density of radioactive substances in them. This in turn makes it possible to precisely determine the location of the hypo- or hyperfunction of a specific organ, which is usually referred to as a cold or a hot artifact.

Unfortunately, the image obtained from a gamma camera is generally not very sharp, as the system of collimators determining from where the recorded radiation came cannot attempt to reach the precision of computed tomography or even an ordinary X-ray. However, if the image is properly filtered (see Fig. 2.46), it can be interpreted by a physician and can form the basis of a good diagnosis.

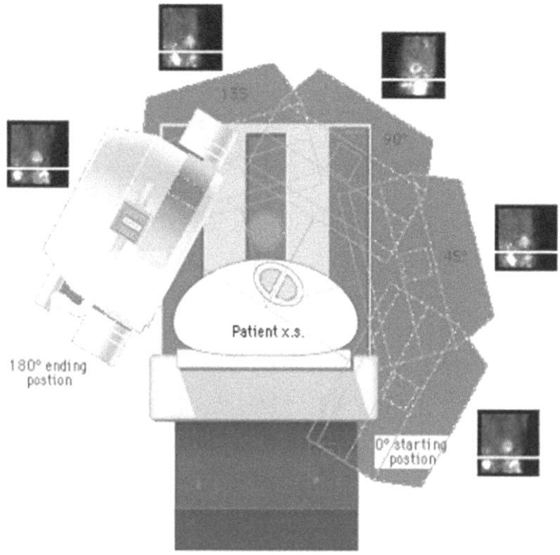

Fig. 2.45. Gamma camera ability to record images from various angles (source Internet)

The organs which are examined using radionuclides (and are the source of the type of images discussed here) mainly include: the thyroid gland (examinations of iodine uptake and metabolism), the heart (the flow of a radionuclide labeled blood allows the degree of ventricle and atrium filling of both parts of the heart to be followed), bones (the skeletal elements in which bone tissue building processes occur, and which are sometimes connected with tumors, can be observed), kidneys (excretion of radioiodinated hipuran) and many others.

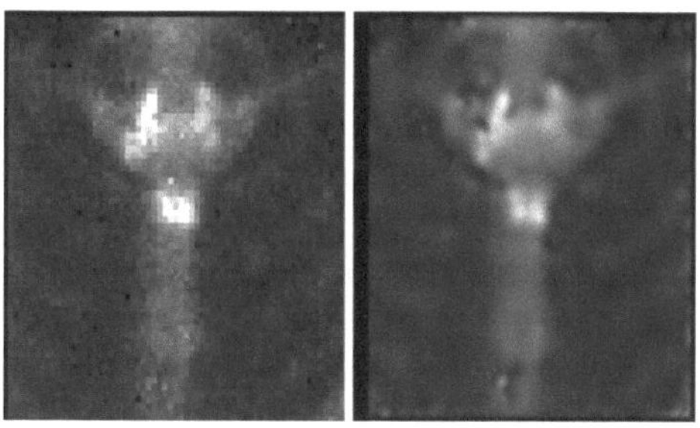

Fig. 2.46. Image from a gamma camera. Unprocessed on the left, filtered on the right

A particularly useful feature of radionuclide examination is that the images produced show not just the static distribution of the concentration of the substance labeled with the radionuclide which is followed in particular parts of the organ, but also the process of accumulating and expulsing that substance from various organs over time (Fig. 2.47). This forms a very valuable source of diagnostic information, which is completely inaccessible in any other way.

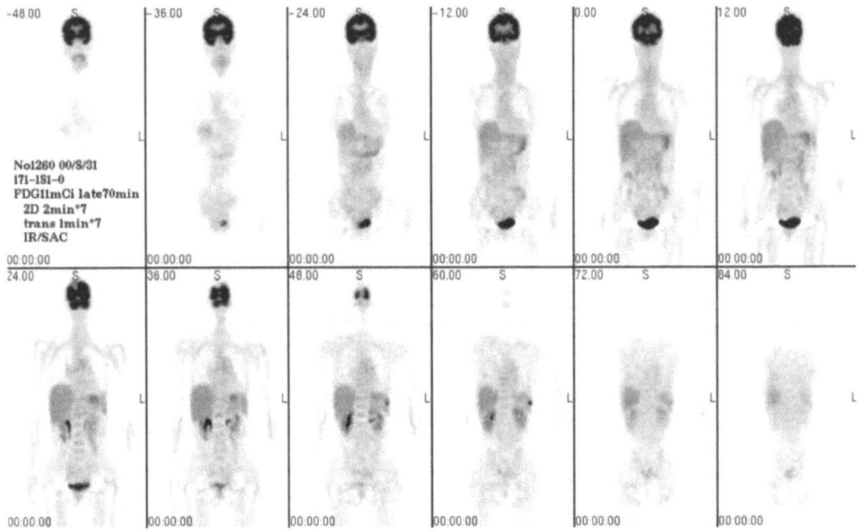

Fig. 2.47. The image of radionuclide distribution within the patient's body, changing over time (source Internet)

2.5. PET imaging

Another modern imaging method called PET (Positron Emission Tomography) is also a radionuclide technique, so in theory it could (or even should) be discussed in the previous chapter. However, as it has many specific characteristics, PET imaging is usually treated as a separate subject, and we will follow that convention in our book [25].

Nowadays, PET is replacing the older and worse technique called SPECT (Single Photon Emission Computed Tomography). PET offers a much better spatial resolution than SPECT and allows one to examine biological events which run much faster. PET makes use of isotopes of much shorter "life", e.g. ^{15}O, ^{13}N and ^{11}C whose half-lifes range from 2 to 20 minutes. Compare this to SPECT, which uses the ^{99m}Tc and ^{127}Xe isotopes with the half-life of 6 hours. This means that a patient undergoing PET examination is examined more precisely and also receives a smaller dose of the harmful radiation. Unfortunately, PET also has a disadvantage: it is extremely expensive!

A diagram of a PET examination is shown in Fig. 2.48. The patient is given a pharmaceutical labeled with a radionuclide of a very short lifetime which for that very reason (as it decays very quickly) cannot be bought for stock, but has to be produced right before the examination in a cyclotron, which forms a part of the PET apparatus set. The interaction between the highly-energetic gamma rays emitted by the isotope and the matter of the human body, causes positrons to be emitted, whose subsequent annihilation is accompanied by the emission of two gamma quanta with the energy of 0.511 MeV in two opposite directions. These events are recorded by a set of detectors distributed around the patient, Fig. 2.49.

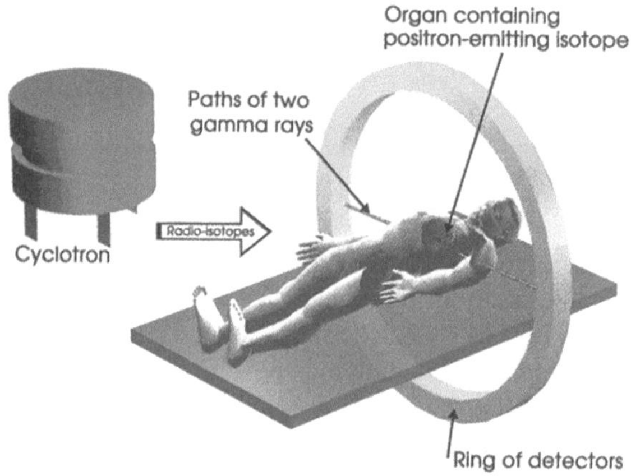

Fig. 2.48. A diagram of a PET imaging apparatus (source Internet)

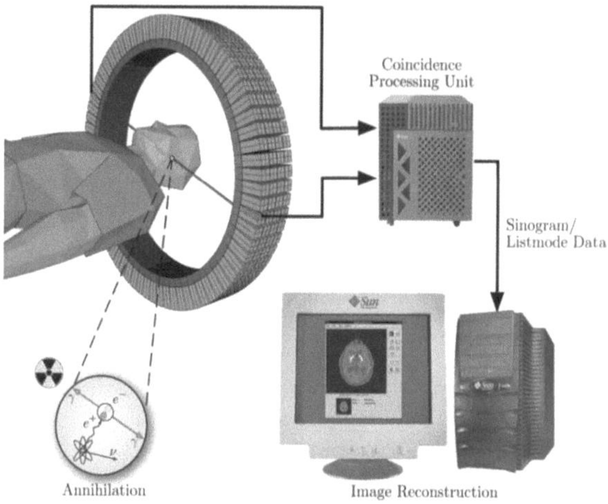

Fig. 2.49. The method of locating the part of the patient's body containing the active atom by capturing the coincidence of two gamma quanta in the ring of detectors (source Internet)

The main advantage of the PET examination is that if fluorodeoxyglucose (FDG) is used to carry the short half-life isotope (fluorine ^{18}F) (Fig. 2.50), the compound ends up in places which at that moment exhibit an increased energy demand, i.e. in areas which are highly active. As the presence and concentration of FDG can be detected with the PET apparatus, it offers an unequalled opportunity to follow the activity of particular organs (mainly the brain).

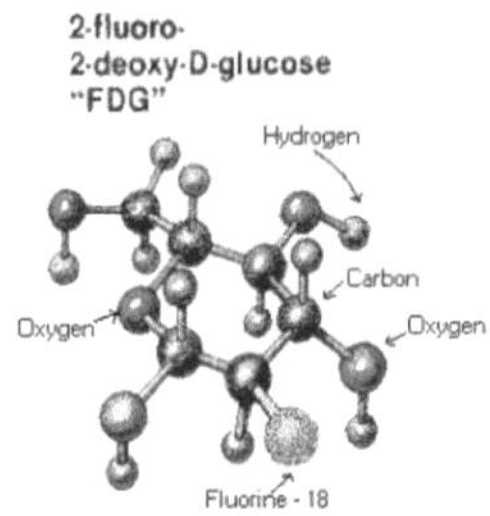

Fig. 2.50. FDG (fluorodeoxyglucose) labeled with the ^{18}F fluorine isotope

A convenient way to follow this is on a series of images showing PET scans of the brain of the same person in four situations: when he/she is intellectually and sensorially inactive (Fig. 2.51), when he/she is solving a math problem (Fig. 2.52), when he/she is watching an interesting picture (Fig. 2.53) and when he/she is listening to a conversation (Fig. 2.54).

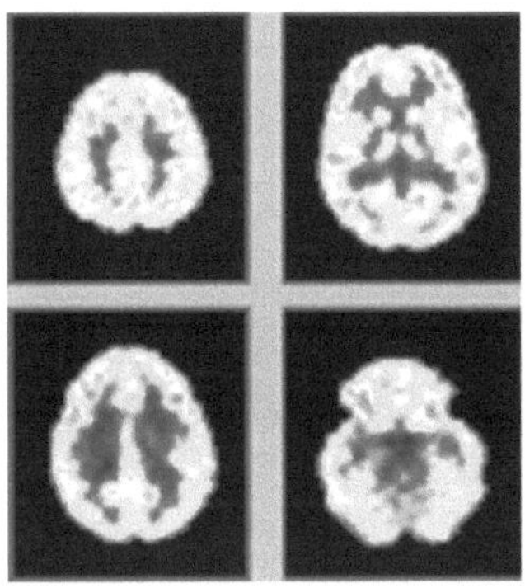

Fig. 2.51. Image of the brain of an awake person who is not concentrating on any specific activity

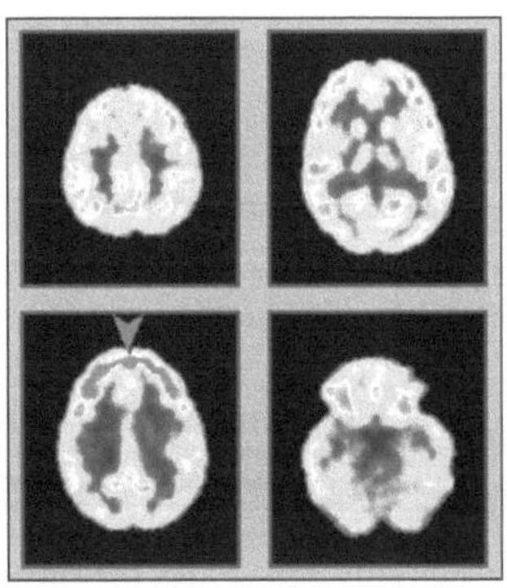

Fig. 2.52. Image of the brain activity of a person solving a difficult math problem. The strong, red color of frontal lobes (indicated by the arrow) shows their activity

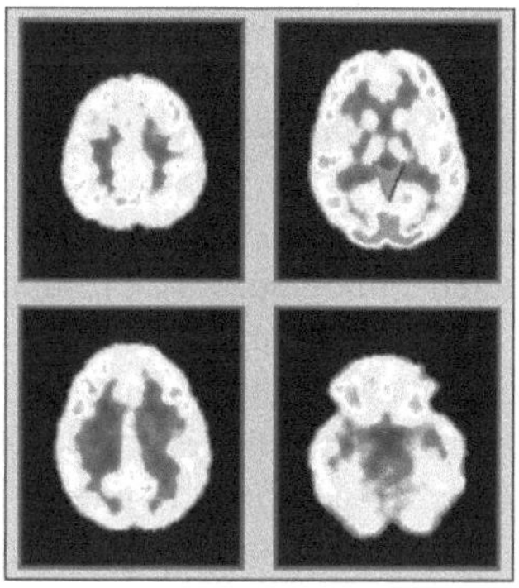

Fig. 2.53. The brain activity of a person watching an interesting scene. A visible activity of occipital lobes which are responsible for receiving and recognizing vision information

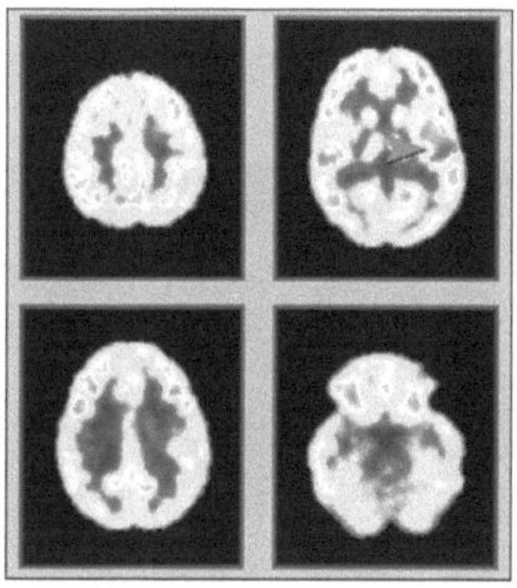

Fig. 2.54. In someone listening to a conversation, activity concentrates in temporal which contain the centers for sound reception and analysis. It is worth noting that temporal areas are active only on one side, as the speech decoding functions are located in only one cerebral hemisphere. If this person were listening to music, both temporal lobes of the brain would "light up".

PET images allow you to record not just the changes in the healthy brain activity connected with the performance of specific activities, but the symptoms of various diseases, as they are very clearly visible in this imaging (Fig. 2.55).

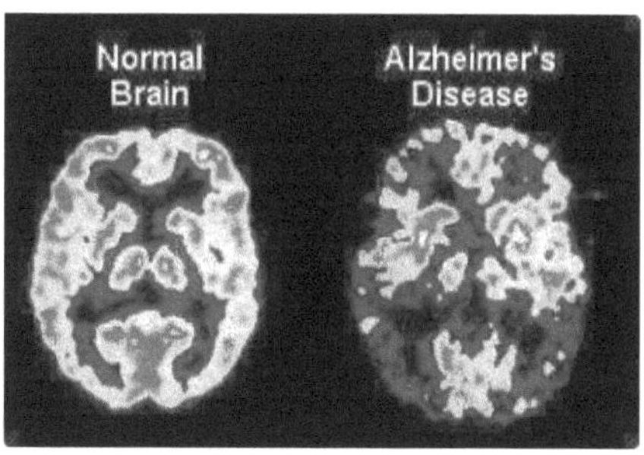

Fig. 2.55. PET images allow lesions to be imaged precisely

One advantage of PET images is that they help to examine the activity of many organs and thus to collect diagnostic information which cannot be acquired in any other way. On the other hand, their shortcoming, obvious in Fig. 2.51–2.54, is the poor resolution for presenting anatomic details. This is why attempts are frequently made to combine the PET image (showing dysfunction locations) with the image from ordinary computed tomography (CT), to get an image rich in both morphological information (identifiable anatomic details, useful for planning and controlling neurosurgical procedures) and in functional information from PET imaging. However, this combination of images is made difficult by problems with the automatic assignment of corresponding fragments of both overlaid images. This is because the CT and PET examinations are made using different apparatuses and at different times, so one cannot expect their cross-section planes to be identical in both images. In addition, both examinations yield images with different resolutions, which necessitates a complex assignment of whole sets of pixels of one image to single pixels of the other. However, a successful overlaying of both images generates an image of exceptional diagnostic and therapeutic utility (Fig. 2.56).

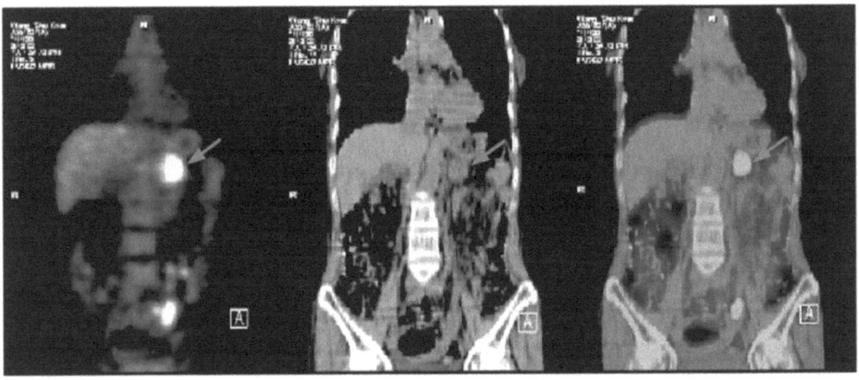

Fig. 2.56. Overlaying PET and CT images. The PET image (left) shows the places in which the function of organs is abnormal, the CT image (middle) shows anatomic details, while the combination of both images (right) gives the best grounds for drawing diagnostic conclusions

2.6. USG images

Ultrasonographic diagnostics (USG) works by emitting recording the reflections of sound waves after they penetrate through tissues and bounce back from boundaries of structures characterized by different densities ρ and different velocities of sound-wave propagation (Fig. 2.57). A short ultrasound impulse sent by the transducer (on the left) propagates through the tissue with the density of ρ_1 and the sound-wave propagation velocity of c_1 and then reaches an organ whose tissues have density ρ_2 and sound-wave propagation velocity c_2. At the boundary between these structures, some of the ultrasound wave is reflected and returns to the ultrasound transducer, creating an echo [4, 5].

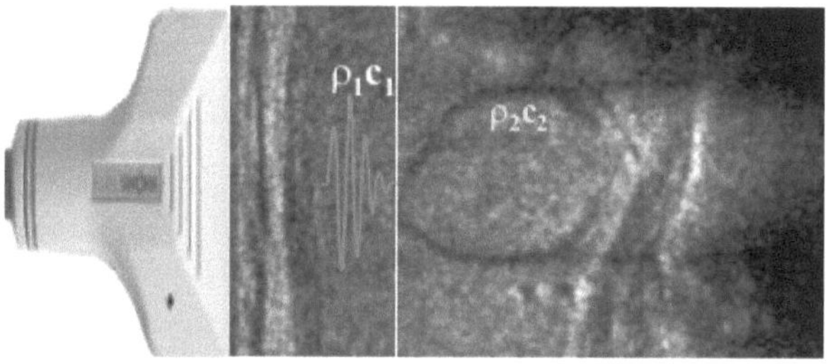

Fig. 2.57. Generation of the ultrasound echo. Described in text

The proportion of the energy of the wave hitting the organ and that reflected from it is determined by the following formula:

$$R = \frac{Z_2 - Z_1}{Z_2 + Z_1} = \frac{\rho_2 c_2 - \rho_1 c_1}{\rho_2 c_2 + \rho_1 c_1}$$

Most frequently, the structures reflecting ultrasound waves are the surfaces of internal organs, whose contours can therefore be detected and located, although sometimes there are reflections from elements within the examined organ which are not distinguished by anything else, producing interference and distortions in the image. The diagram of an USG apparatus is shown in Fig. 2.58.

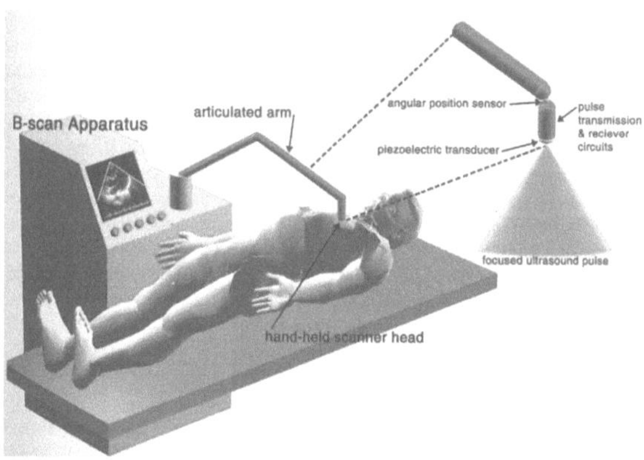

Fig. 2.58. A diagram of the USG apparatus design (source Internet)

The velocities of ultrasound waves in various media are shown in the table 2.1.

Table 2.1. Velocities of ultrasound waves in various media

Substance	Velocity [m/s]
air	340
blood	1,570
bone	2,500 – 4,700
fat	1,450
brain	1,540
liver	1,550
kidney	1,560
spleen	1,578
water	1,530

What is notable is the very large difference in the velocity at which ultrasounds travel through the air and through body tissues. If a layer of air remained between the ultrasound transducer and the patient's skin, 90% of the wave energy would be reflected and would not penetrate the body. This is why, during the examination, the contact between the transducer and the patient's body is so crucial, so to secure it a special gel or water-filled plastic bags are used.

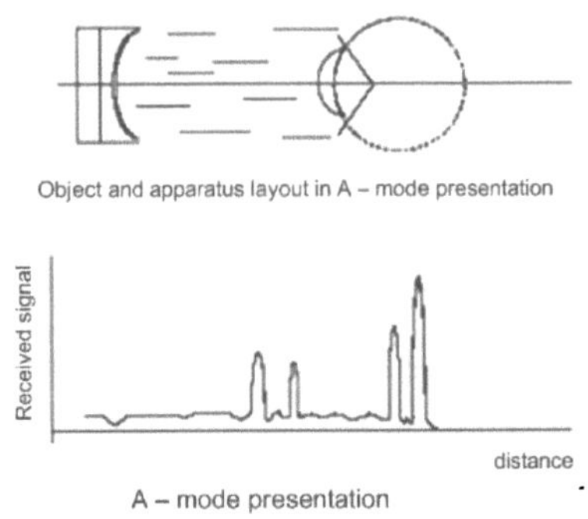

Fig. 2.59. The A presentation of USG examination results

In some cases, immersion examination is conducted in a water bath. All these measures aim at eliminating even the smallest air bubbles from the space between the transducer and the patient's body, as those could disturb the read-out. An alternative examination is intra-operative ultrasonography, done during surgical procedures. This consists in sliding a sterile transducer directly over the examined organ and is very useful in searching for stones in gall ducts or kidneys and for assessing the cancer process [4, 5].

There are several methods for imaging internal organs with the use of the USG. We will discuss them in sequence, indicating their possible uses and the problems connected with the computer transformation of these images.

- The A-mode (Amplitude) presentation is the oldest imaging method in which the piezoelectric transducer generated only short impulses. The whole apparatus operated as an ultrasound echoscope. The echoes of reflected waves, after their amplification in the receiver, were transmitted to the vertical deflection systems of an oscilloscope tube. The time until the echo return was presented on the horizontal axis, which could be calibrated as the scale of the distance from the transducer based on the known ultrasound propagation velocity. A line was plotted above that time/distance axis, and its vertical deflections corresponded to the location of structures reflecting the ultrasound wave (Fig. 2.59). The measurement of the time passing between the return of subsequent echoes was used to determine the position and dimensions of the organs examined (Fig. 2.60). The A-mode presentation had its specific advantages. Experienced physicians (diagnosticians) could determine, on the basis of the slope of the rise and fall of the echo wave, the characteristics of the tissues from which the wave bounced. However, in general, that method provided little information and has since been almost completely discontinued. This examination is only used in a few areas of medicine, including ophthalmology.

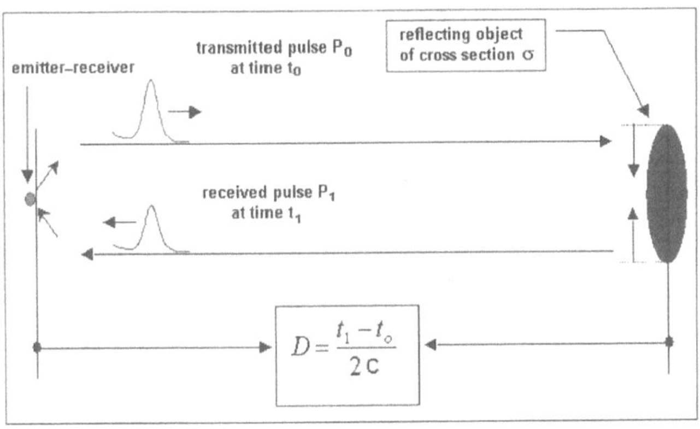

Fig. 2.60. Methods of measuring the location and dimensions of objects in USG examinations

- The B-mode (Brightness) presentation consists in displaying a two-dimensional cross-section of the examined part of the body (e.g. the abdominal cavity) in which the momentary value of the received signal modulates the brightness of subsequent image points. This is based on transforming the amplitude of echoes received from the direction in which the ultrasound beam is propagated into the brightness with which dots shine, as a result of which the monitor shows a line of various brightness. If the ultrasound transceiver is slid and another impulse is sent, the brightened dots will plot another echo line on the monitor. Their character corresponds to the acoustic properties of the part of the organ which is probed with the subsequent ultrasound beam. By repeating this process frequently enough, e.g. by shifting the beam by a distance corresponding to that between adjacent pixels of the monitor (usually the beam is shifted by a distance of several pixels), you get a two-dimensional picture made up of nearby lines of modulated brightness. The structure of the layout of lines making up the B image is usually a fan, due to the design of modern transceivers which usually transmit and receive many ultrasound beams at the same time.

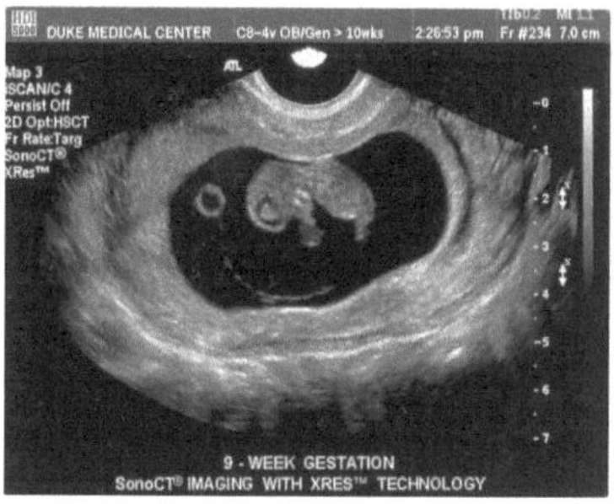

Fig. 2.61. Example of a B-mode sonogram (source Internet)

This technique is frequently used to examine stationary organs. In this method, ultrasound echoes are displayed on the monitor in such a way that they make up a picture of the geometric outline of the examined organ. As the brightness of the dot is proportional to the amplitude of the reflected wave, the organs examined are called more or less echogenic, which term derives from this technique. The horizontal dimension of the dot depends on the width of the echo at its base. The bigger the echo, the brighter the dot. B-mode USG images are usually saved with the resolution of 700×500 pixels or lower and a brightness depth represented with 8 bits. An example image obtained by the B-mode presentation is shown in Fig. 2.61. By superposing a number of B-mode images one over the other using a computer, a 3D image of a very realistic appearance (Fig. 2.62) can be obtained, which is frequently very useful, although by no means necessary for the diagnostic suitability of the image.

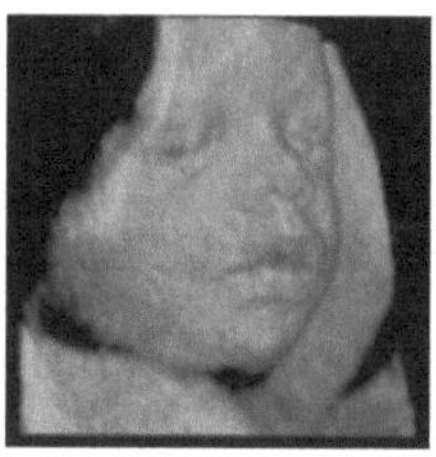

Fig. 2.62. A 3D reconstruction of an object (the fetus's head in its mother's womb) obtained by a computer processing of a B-mode presentation

- **M**-mode **(M**otion**)** presentation, formerly called **TM** (**T**ime **M**otion), consists in listening to the echo from the same direction at two subsequent moments. The echoes are displayed as in the B-mode, which means that the momentary value of the signal modulates the brightness of the dots displayed, and subsequent lines are drawn vertically side by side. In this option, the time base of the oscilloscopic tube brightens only in the places where ultrasound echoes appear. Echoes coming from mobile organs are represented on the time base by mobile bright dots, which leave a trace on the screen. The M-mode presentation is still fundamental in examining the function and imaging the structure of the heart (Fig. 2.63). Its other uses include imaging the abdominal aorta, and in particular its aneurisms.

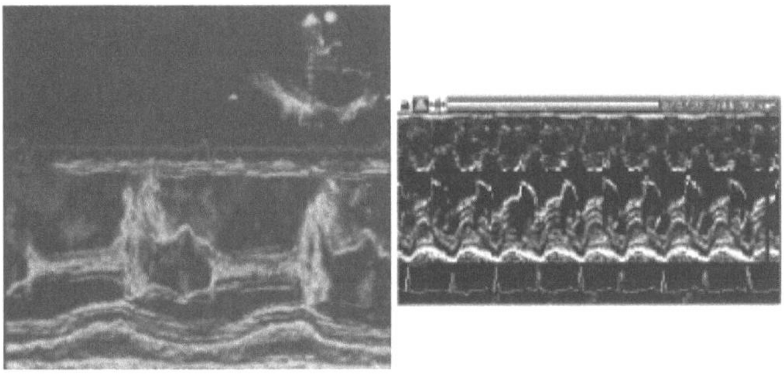

Fig. 2.63. An M-mode USG image

- The **D**-mode **(D**oppler**)** consists in receiving the USG wave dispersed by the moving blood cells, which returns to the transceiver with a changed frequency (the Doppler effect). Depending on the velocity and direction of blood cell motion relative to the USG beam and the direction in which the wave is propagated, there is a Doppler shift of the frequency of the sent and received wave towards higher or lower frequencies. On the image, this is usually shown in color: blue for the fastest movement in one direction, and red for the fastest motion in the opposite direction. Intermediate colors code movements at lower velocities, while the echoes coming from stationary structures are presented as black-and-white. An example of a very beautiful D-mode image is shown in Fig. 2.64. It presents the umbilical cord of a fetus.

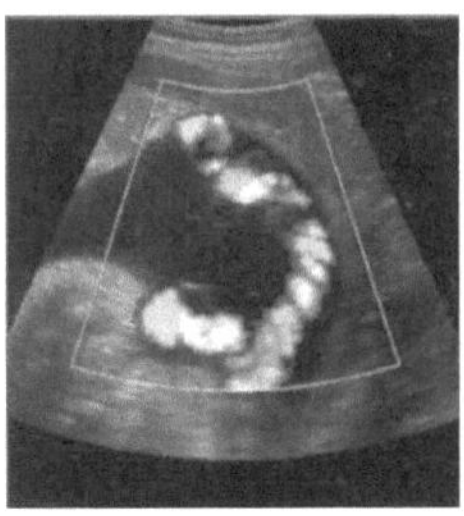

Fig. 2.64. An image obtained by D-mode presentation

Obviously, the umbilical cord channels the flow in two directions, as the intertwined blood vessels transport blood to and from the placenta – which is very clear in the image. The D-mode presentation is used to diagnose the blood flow, one purpose of which can be to locate narrowings of blood vessels, and therefore constitutes a key diagnostic tool in modern cardiology. The technique has the following varieties:

- The **CFM-mode** (Color Flow Mapping) presentation consists in filling a sector of the B-mode black-and-white image selected by the operator with a color image of the flows measured using the correlation technique.
- The **CFA-mode** (Color Flow Angiography) consists in identifying the flow, assigning a color to the areas in which the flow has been identified and incorporating them in the black and white B-mode image.

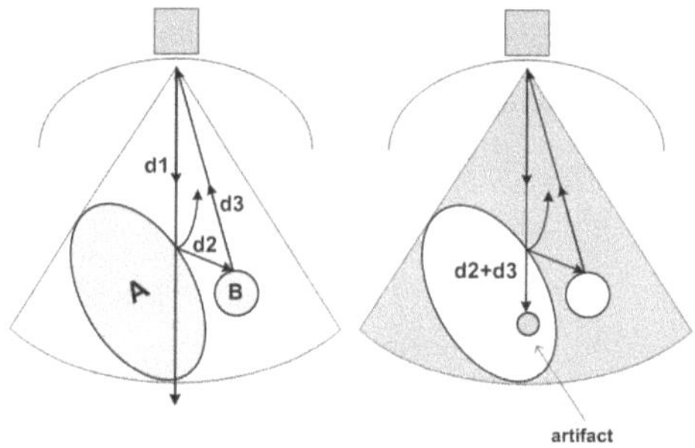

Fig. 2.65. Creating artifacts in a USG image

The USG image may be subject to much more noises and deformations that other medical images described previously here. There are many causes of deformations. The simplest one is called specles. This is a non-uniform structure of the ultrasonographic image caused by the local interference of waves reflected within the medium. Specles look like randomly distributed black and grey spots on the bright image background. They depend on the non-uniformity of the medium and the magnitude of impulses probing it. Another source of noise consists of the different velocities at which ultrasound travels through layers of tissues which make it difficult to precisely scale the dimensions of the examined structures. As we know, the USG apparatus measures the differences in the return time of the echo bouncing from different structures and presents them on the image under the assumption that the distance traveled by the impulse over a unit of time is the same in every place, which is obviously untrue. What is more, the surfaces between environments of various ultrasound propagation velocities not only reflect waves (which is necessary to obtain the image), but also refract them. As a result, the probing impulses, instead of traveling down straight lines along the direction of the beam produced, which is assumed when generating the USG image, follow an indeterminate, winding and complicated route, which can only be roughly approximated as a straight line. The dampening of the energy of the wave penetrating tissues weakens the echoes returning from deeper structures, as a result of which the image is darker behind structures which reflect a lot (an acoustic shadow appears). All the above phenomena disturb the image and cause artifacts to appear – Fig. 2.65. Artifacts appear in the USG image as the echoes of objects which:

1. Do not really exist (multiple reflections);
2. Are represented in the wrong location (multiple reflections, wave refraction);
3. Are of deformed dimensions, shape and brightness (wave refraction, phase aberration, various sound velocities).

The majority of artifacts are caused by the physical properties of wave propagation through tissues, but some are caused by the incorrect setting of the apparatus, mainly the amplification, the range adjustment of amplification as well as the pre- and post-processing functions selected [4, 5].

3. Compressing medical images and storing them in medical databases

3.1. Systems for archiving and distributing medical images

The consideration of various types of medical images cannot focus only on the technical aspects of their acquisition, processing, analysis and recognition (which will be the subject of further considerations), but should analyze the ways in which they are used. Medical images are obviously acquired mainly for diagnostic reasons, so we write a lot about the ways of making a good use of computer image analysis as a tool supporting the diagnostic process in this book. Images are sometimes also used to aid therapy, one example being Intensity-Modulated Radiation Therapy (IMRT).

So a digital image is an important, and actually an increasingly important item in the documentation of the patient and his/her disease, leading to the appearance of new IT duties. It is no wonder that medical images are currently handled by all IT systems operated by healthcare units. Such systems are usually orientated towards acquiring, archiving and transmitting medical images complemented with all the necessary data on the patient and his/her medical history.

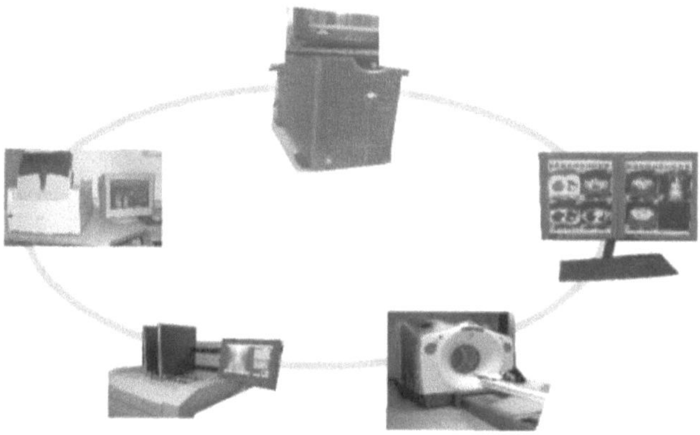

Fig. 3.1. An example structure of an older generation PACS system with a separate FDDI ring for fast image transfer (source Internet)

The widespread installation of medical imaging apparatuses delivering images in a digital format (in particular CT and MRI scanners) in 1980s, when the benefits of storing data on digital media became obvious, mark the beginnings of the rapid development of PACS (Picture Archiving and Communication Systems), which still continues today. These systems support archiving, transferring and accessing medical images and represent modern counterparts of traditional archives

M.R. Ogiela and R. Tadeusiewicz: *Compressing medical images and stroring them in medical databases,* Studies in Computational Intelligence (SCI) **84**, 47–63 (2007)
www.springerlink.com

of exposed plates. Such systems are used for either long- or short-term storage of images acquired using various methods of medical imaging, as well as for transmitting such images for remote diagnostics or consultations.

As it was necessary to rapidly transmit large files of data, which medical images always represent, the first structures of PACS systems were based on the assumption that the exchange and circulation of this image information would run over a separate structure of very fast communication elements, such as an FDDI ring (Fig. 3.1). Sources of image signals (e.g. computed tomography apparatuses) were connected to that ring, as were devices for viewing, analyzing and saving medical images, and that ring was not directly integrated with other elements of the hospital computer network.

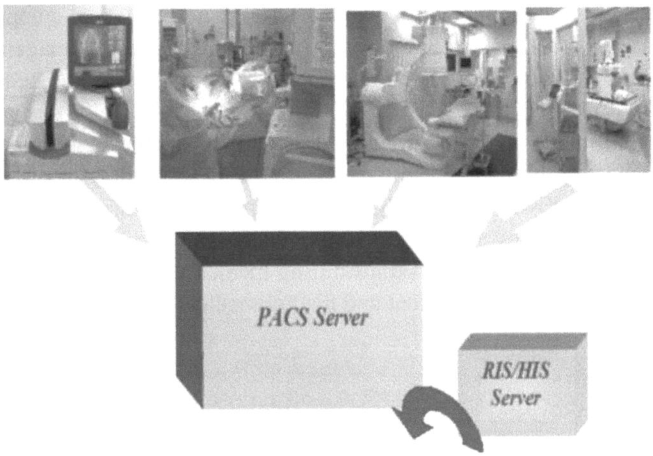

Fig. 3.2. A PACS system integrated with the hospital system (source Internet)

Nowadays, PACS systems are increasingly frequently integrated with RIS systems (Radiological Information Systems) which represent the radiology part of the Hospital Information System (HIS), which in turn stores patients' data and radiology reports in the text format (Fig. 3.2). Obviously, to streamline the handling of medical images (whose volume keeps rising with every next generation of medical apparatuses), special servers are installed to handle the image part of the system. This is the standard situation today, but as the computing power of ordinary workstations with which hospitals are equipped keeps rising along with the growing capacity of standard components of typical computer networks, the historical isolation of the PACS system from the rest of the IT hospital hardware has actually been overcome. It seems that medical records with which we will increasingly deal at clinics and other health care institutions in the future will be of multimedia nature (see Fig. 3.3), combining images and text elements of the documentation into modern multimedia structures managed and handled by integrated hospital information systems.

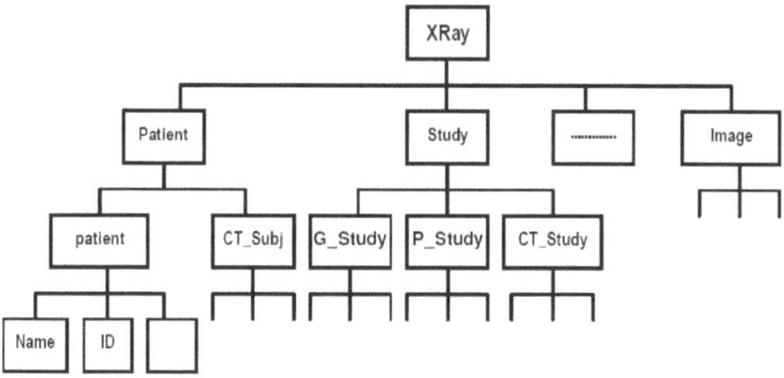

Fig. 3.3. A typical structure of a multimedia patient record

A PACS server may also provide image data simultaneously to many workstations, to printers producing the documentation, and to diagnostic stations, and also disseminate this data externally via a network (Fig. 3.4). This ensures immediate access to the complete information about the patient, both textual, including examination results in the form of tables of numbers, and image information, at any time and place, also over portable wireless devices. These solutions became widespread due to the improved methods of medical image compression discussed further on in this chapter.

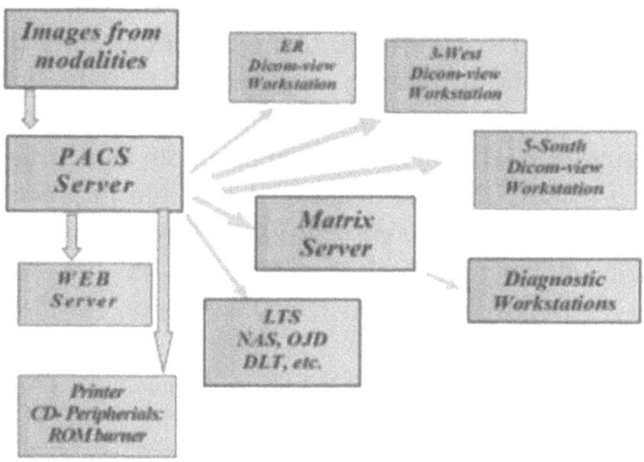

Fig. 3.4. The role of a PACS system as the distributor of medical images

3.2. Standards for medical images treated as computer data files

As a rule, files generated by medical imaging systems contain images (in the original or compressed format), patient's identification and demographic data as well as technical information on the examination itself. At the beginning, individual manufacturers of medical apparatuses (General Electric, Siemens, Philips, Picker, Hitachi, Shimadzu, Toshiba, Elscint, Imatron) used proprietary formats for saving data (and sometimes even non-standard storage media), frequently different for different image types. However, along with the development of the aforementioned PACS systems, frequently running not just in a single hospital but also making use of Wide Area Networks (WAN), standardization became necessary.

The first notable standard format for storing and transmitting images was ACR/NEMA 1.0 and 2.0 developed by the American College of Radiologists (ACR) and the National Electrical Manufacturers Association (NEMA). The first published version of this standard was announced in 1985 in a document entitled ACR/NEMA S.P. No. 300-1985, which is currently referred to as ACR/NEMA 1.0. That version had relatively limited capabilities, but it became the kernel around which subsequent system versions could be built, including version 2.0 in 1988. In 1992 and 1993, there were further publications dealing with the ACR/NEMA 3.0 standard, whose supplementing lasted for as long as until 2001. After many modifications, which never compromised back compatibility, the ACR/NEMA format became the current **DICOM 3** standard described in greater detail lower down in this chapter. One can assume that the majority of systems for medical data acquisition, transmission and storage currently developed worldwide complies with that standard [16].

ACR/NEMA was not the only proposal of a universal standard. However, the other ones, like Papyrus, Interfile V3.3, Qsh and DEFF have not gained much popularity. DICOM 3 overtook them and is currently the unquestioned universal standard, as from the very beginning it was designed to be a constantly evolving standard. So if new medical apparatuses introduce a new quality of imaging (e.g. 3D images), the appropriate data structures are immediately reflected in DICOM, but to make it possible to process the new data also using older medical processing and interpretation applications, the modifications introduced must be back compatible with previous versions. The most up to date officially published DICOM version (at the time of writing this book) is PS 3-2004.

Compared to ACR/NEMA, DICOM 3 introduces a number of enhancements. It defines, among other things:

- the communication method in the TCP/IP network environment (ACR/NEMA defined only the communication protocol in a point-point environment);
- data storage methods (types of physical media and logical file systems);
- the method of data exchange and the syntax of instructions sent between devices (including the notion of service classes);
- the notion of the information object for various types of data.

The general structure of the DICOM network protocol is presented on Fig. 3.5.

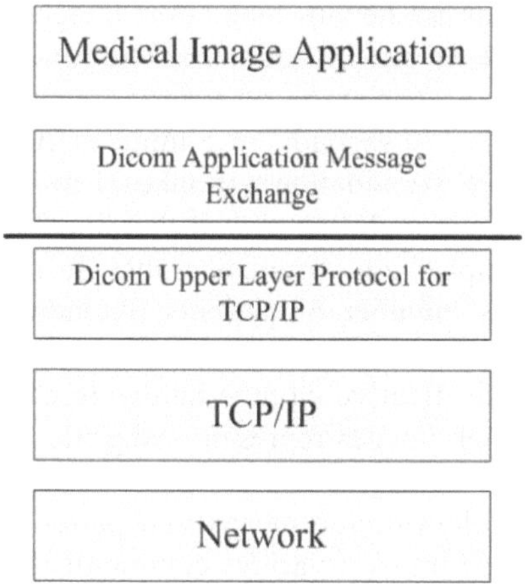

Fig. 3.5. Network architecture of the DICOM protocol

3.3. Why medical images need to be compressed

The decision to record, archive and transmit medical images in the digital format immediately required selecting the appropriate technique for compressing them, as an uncompressed medical image in the form in which it is generated by a CT apparatus, for example, is represented in the digital system by a data file of a huge volume: dozens and sometimes even hundreds of megabytes. Compression helps to cut this volume between several and over a dozen times, so after compression, images can be stored at a lower cost. Let us make a short illustrative calculation:

A typical mammography examination made as part of a screening program produces two images of each breast in the cranio-caudal and transverse projections. Each of these images is 40 MB (megabytes) of data on the average, which represents: 4*40 M = 160 MB of data from every examination. If uncompressed, the results of just 3 or 4 such examinations can be written to a 700 MB CD, while in a typical screening programmer, the results for at least several hundred patients need to be recorded. The problems of collecting and storing this data and also of accessing them efficiently, including quickly finding them when they are needed becomes a daunting organizational problem. Bear in mind that this data has to be stored for at least 10 years!

Let's consider the same problem from a different perspective. In a clinical environment, a radiology lab conducts some 30 image examinations a day on the average. This means that the hospital database receives 30*160 MB = 4.8 GB of data a day. How long will it take to exhaust the disk storage resources of even a very large server?

Or from another perspective. Let's say that we need to consult a mammography examination case with a specialist from another hospital or another city.

We get in touch, agree that he/she will look at the image and assess it, we start sending the image ... and we get in trouble, as the time needed to transmit a single mammogram over a connection of a very good speed (by today standards) equal to 1 Mbit/s is 320 seconds, or 5 minutes 20 seconds, while sending the results of the entire examination will take 21 minutes 20 seconds. Will our expert have the good will and time to wait that long?

So medical image compression is indispensable. It means that the medical documentation of a large number of patients, including numerous medical images, can be stored on the storage media available at present (e.g. a RAID disk array) or that a more cost effective storage hardware can be designed for the hospital IT system in which images represent a significant share of the patient documentation recorded and analyzed.

The development of telemedicine means that patient information increasingly frequently has to be sent over various communication channels. Medical image compression clearly can help here, as compressed images can not only be collected more effectively, but are also easier and less expensive to transmit over ICT connections when it becomes necessary to consult remotely.

Systems which archive medical image data can use various techniques for data compression, depending on the requirements to be met by the fidelity of image recovery after compression and also depending on whether the data is in the form of static images or visualizations of moving objects (e.g. the parts of a beating heart). We will try to briefly review the related issues.

3.4. General remarks about image compression methods

Most generally, image compression can be divided into two types: **lossy** and **lossless.**

According to information theory, lossless compression only removes the redundancy (redundant information) present in the image or other data being compressed. Lossy compression, on the other hand, also removes parts of material information (material from the point of view of information theory and the ability to recreate the original image structure) in addition to the redundancy. If high ratios of lossy compression are used, they may cause a significant loss of the information originally present.

The above names indicate that if lossless compression is used, a previously compressed image can be recovered in and will be no different at all from the original. Of course, we have to use the appropriate decompression algorithm for that purpose, but lossless compression leads to no information loss.

If lossy compression is used, we accept that a certain proportion of information contained in the original picture will be irrecoverably lost. It may sound somewhat scary. A picture coded using a lossy compression method cannot be recovered in its original form, and some details of the objects which were visible in the original picture will not be visible in a picture which has been compressed and then recovered. This characteristic of lossy compression techniques meant that for many years, lossy compression of medical images was out of the question, as their contents could determine the diagnosis, and the diagnosis could mean the difference the life and death of the patient.

Today, this radical view has been moderated. It should be emphasized that image features "lost" during a properly conducted lossy compression are mainly those that are not well perceived by the human eye anyway. For example, the JPEG algorithm, one of the best known algorithms for lossy image compression, loses mainly high-frequency image changes along the diagonal (45° to the vertical or horizontal direction). These changes are almost unperceivable to the human eye, so subjectively, when we look at the original picture and the picture subjected to lossy compression, we can see no significant difference.

Consequently, if the optimum compression ratio is selected, the information loss occurring during the compression of typical images is so small as to be unnoticeable, or if it is noticeable, it is negligible and leads to only an insignificant reduction in picture quality. If the image quality loss is so negligible that it is not perceivable due to the imperfections of human sight, the algorithm is popularly referred to as "visually lossless".

On the other hand, the benefits are huge, as lossy compression methods allow the information volume of an image to be reduced many times more than even the best lossless compression methods. This means that when there is a need to significantly reduce the size of images, visually lossy compression must usually be used, regardless of its shortcomings.

Consequently, the following compromise is accepted for medical images today:

Less sensitive medical images (e.g. those produced during screening tests) are compressed with lossy algorithms which yield compression rates better than lossless algorithms. Lossy compression can be used in this case also for the reason that physicians give these images a cursory glance, only looking for large and clear pathological symptoms in them, and not for some hard to see subtleties.

In contrast, images used in the sensitive and difficult process of diagnostics are compressed using only lossless compression methods, which are also preferred for archiving images that are to form comparative documentation allowing one to follow the development of the disease process or the progress of the treatment and rehabilitation process in the future.

Important arguments against using lossy compression methods for medical images include:

- The loss of material information during lossy compression occurs even for low compression ratios. Only negligible values of this ratio cause no noticeable losses in the quality of images or losses of significant information;

- A low degree of lossy compression, which leads to moderate distortion, also yields mediocre results in terms of information reduction compared to the improved methods of lossless compression;
- There are problems in defining the future quality requirements for images currently compressed in a lossy way. This may be important if images are to be stored for a long time;
- There is no optimum measure for assessing a lossy compression algorithm or to define its ratio that would be suitable for assessing the compression quality of medical images used for diagnostic purposes. Measure systems like Peak Signal to Noise Ratio (PSNR) cannot be said to be consistent with subjective image quality assessments made by observers, or to be consistent with results achieved by observers when analysing images compressed in a lossy way;
- Visually lossless algorithms may not always turn out to be diagnostically lossless. Attempts as assessing whether an image is diagnostically lossless may be of very limited utility due to the variable perception of the human sight.
- Methods of automatic image interpretation may be sensitive (from the point of view of the effectiveness of final diagnosis) to changes caused by lossy compression;
- There are difficulties in performing adaptive compression, i.e. compressing image areas important for diagnostics with lower ratios and compressing areas which contain no diagnostic information with higher ratios.

All the above problems illustrate the problems that can be caused by applying compression methods to archive medical data. No such problems are encountered if lossless techniques are used, but such algorithms usually feature relatively lower ratios of reduction of the space occupied by the image.

3.5. Lossless compression methods

Lossless compression methods achieve their result, i.e. reduce the information volume of a picture, due to the fact (in the simplest case) that two adjacent pixels of a medical image are frequently of the same value. For example, if there is a background pixel in a specific part of an X-ray image as the image of the examined body part is visible elsewhere, the pixels adjacent to that pixel are very likely to also represent the background and be of exactly the same grey level – Fig. 3.6.

And so, instead of recording the same value many times for many pixels of the image, the value can be recorded only once with information added that this value is repeated in a given line of the image a hundred times, for example. Such groups of adjacent pixels of exactly the same grey level can, of course, be found in all parts of the analyzed image (for example within the visible bones), although as a rule, the greatest gain is achieved by the abbreviated coding of groups of background pixels.

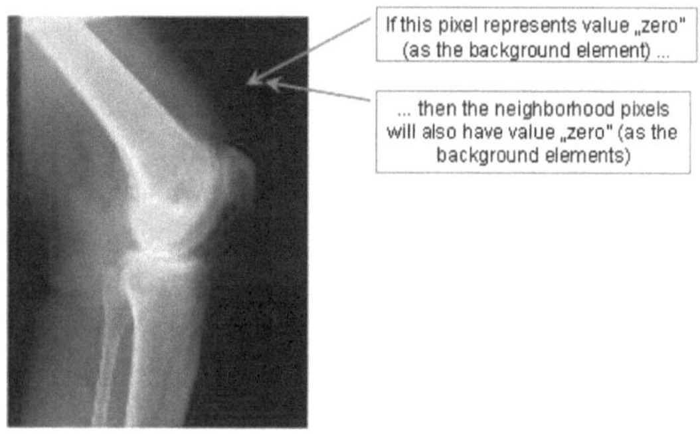

Fig. 3.6. The simplest method of lossless compression consists in the abbreviated coding of groups of pixels with the same grey level

Another simple idea for achieving lossless image compression is the so called entropic coding. Without reference to the rather complex mathematical methodology of this transformation, which is by and large connected to elements of the Shannon information theory, it can be generally said that this compression is based on using various numbers of bits to code various grey levels of pixels in the image. In the original image obtained from the medical imaging apparatus, every pixel is coded with the same number of bits, resulting from the selected resolution of the grey scale of the image. The typical resolution is one byte per pixel, but some examinations (like CT) generate images in which pixels values are expressed with 12 bits. In the compressed image, the number of bits linked with different grey levels is highly differentiated. In general, the less frequent the grey level in the picture, the longer coding word can describe it – Fig. 3.7.

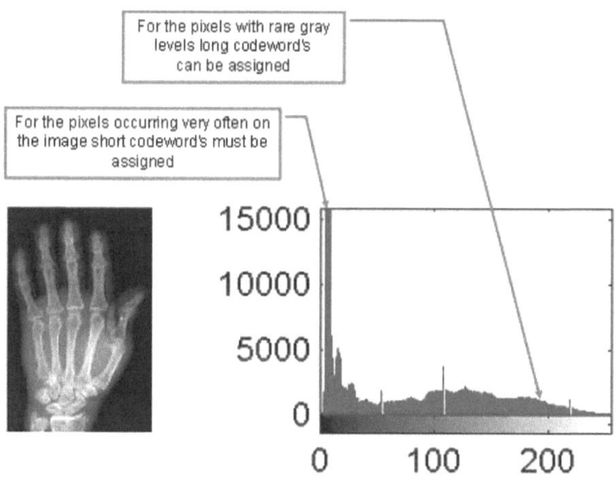

Fig. 3.7. Medical image (left) and its histogram (right). The principle of entropy coding means assigning short code words to relatively frequent image pixels (tall bars in the histogram) and longer code words to rare pixels

To start compressing with the method described here, we first search (usually using the histogram – see Fig. 3.7) for the value of pixels which are the most frequent in the picture (usually the pixels of the large image background are the most frequent) and we use a very short code, sometimes of as little as only one byte, to code these grey levels. Then, we use somewhat longer code words to represent the pixels which are somewhat less frequent, but still more widespread than others. The rule described above indicates that long code words will be few, while the majority of pixels will be described with short code words. In total, the number of bits needed to describe the entire picture can be significantly cut, which is the advantage of this method of coding.

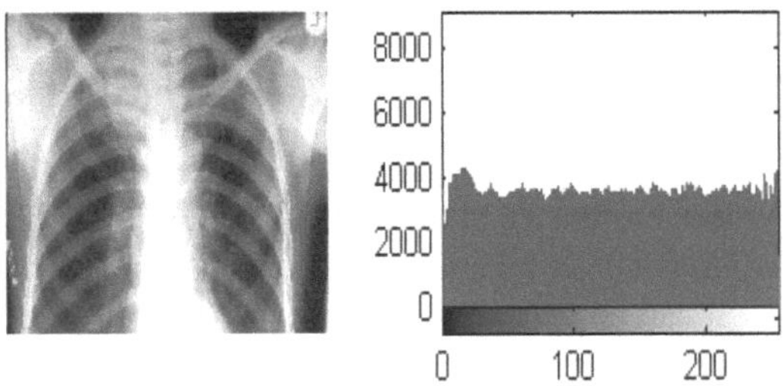

Fig. 3.8. A medical image with little variation in its histogram is difficult to compress with entropy coding.

The above principle of lossless entropy coding is simplified compared to the actual algorithms used, but it gives the reader an idea of why the same picture can be recorded using much fewer bits (in total), while the original picture can always be precisely recovered keeping all the details it originally contained. However, it should be noted that not all medical images have such a varied frequency of pixels of various brightness (cf. Fig. 3.8), so entropy coding may sometimes fail to live up to our expectations.

More advanced lossless compression algorithms use prediction methods. In these algorithms the data (i.e. the pixel value) to be encoded at present is predicted based on nearby data (usually that closest in the space of the picture and therefore potentially the most correlated with it), which has already appeared in the sequence being encoded. The encoding algorithm makes a strict and unchangeable connection between the sequence of previous pixels and the value of the pixel being "guessed at". This is essential for the causality condition, necessary to reconstruct the source image during the decoding. Only the imprecision of the prediction is encoded.

A prediction coding method on which practical implementations are based is referred to as DPCM (differential pulse code modulation). The beginnings of DPCM methods can be traced to work done at Bell Laboratories. Their significant limitation is due to the imperfection of prediction, whose causes include the impossibility of creating the context (neighborhood) of prediction surrounding the coded pixel on every side (the need to observe the causality condition).

HINT (hierarchical interpolation) algorithms represent a modified prediction method in which the encoding/decoding of subsequent versions of the image of higher and higher resolutions are used. Due to this, the values of pixels surrounding the pixel on each side, but not always closest to it, are used for predictions. The differential images obtained from the prediction are usually coded using the Huffman or arithmetic code.

3.6. Compression standards

Compression standards applied in PACS systems frequently include lossy algorithms and hybrid ones, i.e. those ones that come in both lossless and lossy varieties.

In the DICOM standard, lossy algorithms can be used almost exclusively to compress motion sequences, where the impact of artifacts brought about by information reduction is much smaller than for static pictures. This is because in motion sequences, the recording standards frequently allow the shapes to be predicted based on information from nearby video frames.

An analysis of topics of research on medical image compression [8, 12] and the DICOM standard [16] indicates that algorithms developed for broad groups of various kinds of images, not just medical, are most frequently used to compress medical images.

The compression techniques used in such systems include:

- Standard Lossless JPEG – a lossless, predictive encoding scheme for images with the brightness depth of 2–16 bits per pixel. The algorithm is a part of the JPEG standard which also includes a lossy algorithm, but both algorithms differ much. The JPEG standard calls for compressing in the raster sequence as well as progressive encoding. One of the elements of the Lossless JPEG algorithm is an entropy encoder, and the JPEG standard calls for using Huffman codes or the arithmetic coder in it.
- FELICS – a simple, fast predictive lossless compression algorithm which achieves moderate compression ratios (though better than Lossless JPEG with a Huffman encoder), in which the entropy encoder is based on the parametric family of Golomb codes;
- BTPC – a lossless, predictive and transformative hierarchical system with an adaptive entropy encoder based on Huffman codes;
- S + P – a predictive and transformative hierarchical scheme with an adaptive entropy coder based on Huffman codes or an arithmetic encoder. The S + P algorithm comes in two forms: lossy and lossless.
- PNG – a standard developed and recommended by the WWW Consortium for color and grey-level images with the brightness depth of up to 16 bits per pixel. PNG is a predictive scheme in which a progressive coding option has also been defined. PNG uses LZ77 dictionary coding with an entropy encoder based on Huffman codes.

- DICOM RLE – a variant of a simple, universal algorithm for sequence length coding designed for coding images losslessy. This variety is a method, taken over by the DICOM standard, previously used to encode TIFF-format images, called TIFF Packbits, designed for images with an 8-bit depth of brightness.
- CALIC – a lossless predictive algorithm [65] considered to represent the gold standard of lossless image compression. It achieves mean compression ratios better than other algorithms. The downside is that it is relatively slow to run. In the CALIC algorithm, the entropy encoder is based on the Huffman algorithm or arithmetic coding.
- JPEG-LS standard – a predictive algorithm for compressing images whose resolution falls within the 2–16 bit/pixel brightness scale. The standard includes two options: a lossless and a lossy one (called near-lossless, in which only small losses are accepted). Just as in the FELICS algorithm, the entropy encoder is based on the parametric family of Golomb codes. The LOCO-I algorithm [62] is the core of the JPEG-LS algorithm
- JPEG2000 standard, which defines, among other items, a progressive coding and transmission scheme as well as lossy and lossless transformative (wavelet transformation) methods for compressing images in steps [12]. JPEG2000 was inspired by the work of CREW algorithm authors [8] which showed the multitude of useful practical features of hierarchical transform algorithms. The core of the JPEG2000 algorithm is based on the EBCOT algorithm [62]. In the JPEG2000 algorithm, the entropy encoder uses arithmetic coding.

3.7. Comparison of compression methods

This subsection compares the above compression methods and presents the ratios achieved by selected algorithms. These results are based on research by David A. Cluine [13], who compared the effectiveness of compression methods using a set of 2922 medical images of RTG, MR, USG and CT types.

Table 3.1 presents compression ratios (CR) of selected algorithms for specific types of medical images. These are defined as the u/c, where u is the size of the uncompressed image in bytes, and c is the size in bytes of that image after compression. The value of that ratio tells us how many times smaller the file containing the image will be after the compression. Table 3.1 shows average compression rates for images of particular types – CT, MR, USG, RTG – as well as the arithmetic mean of these values representing the average compression rate of each algorithm.

Table 3.1. Comparison of compression rates achieved for selected medical image types by several selected algorithms for lossless image compression

Algorithm	Image type				
	CT	MR	USG	RTG	Mean
S + P(H)	3.19	3.15	1.52	2.16	2.51
PNG	2.64	2.54	3.04	2.18	2.60
S + P(A)	3.72	3.71	1.68	2.28	2.85
Standard Lossless JPEG	3.29	2.97	2.38	2.76	2.85
JPEG2000	3.88	3.63	2.97	3.14	3.41
CALIC(H)	3.79	3.59	3.20	3.12	3.43
JPEG-LS	4.00	3.59	3.39	3.15	3.53
CALIC(A)	4.01	3.72	3.50	3.23	3.62

This comparison shows that the algorithm which currently achieves the best compression rates for medical (and other) images is CALIC(A). Unfortunately, it is very slow, so it is rarely used in practice, just treated as a reference or an indicator of the lossless compression ratios that can be achieved.

In practice, the JPEG-LS and JPEG2000 algorithms allow the size of a file containing a medical image to be reduced several times while retaining all the data. Depending on the type of image, the compression rates of these algorithms range from 3 to 4, with the average of about 3.5. Older algorithms, such as LJPG and PNG perform somewhat worse than JPEG-LS or JPEG2000 in this comparison, while universal compression algorithms and DICOM RLE are the worst.

It is easy to notice that individual types of medical images are characterized by differences in compression rates big enough to make some algorithms potentially better for some image types, while others are better for other images. This is due to the nature of the lossless compression process. In this compression, certain characteristics of the compressed image are used (e.g. the fact that series of pixels with the same value occur next to each other). If a given type of medical images exhibits this feature frequently and for large pixel groups, then these images can be compressed very well with this algorithm. However, if the medical image has features much different from those taken into account when developing the compression method, then compressing it using this type of an algorithm will not yield good results. This is obvious for some algorithms when one looks at Table 3.1.

On the other hand, if the differences in results generated by selected algorithms for different image types are negligible, this means that the algorithm uses characteristics and features present in very many different images. This is good for designers of medical imaging systems, as then an algorithm yielding a very good compression rate for one medical type will also achieve a very good ratio for other types, so the designers can use it for every file containing an image without considering the method by which it was acquired.

The compression rate achieved using a given image archiving technique is of major practical significance, but the development of compression methods shows that this is not the only or decisive factor. Actually, one of the key factors which determine the potential application of a specific compression algorithm in the given medical imaging system is the availability of standards that support using it to uniformly process images acquired by apparatuses of various manufacturers. Standardizing methods for compressing and representing medical images also supports data exchange between those apparatuses, and simplifies data management and its uniform processing by different programs as there is no need to use separate programs for filtering and de-noising various images, applying universal algorithms supporting such standards instead.

In medical applications, the algorithms most frequently used to losslessly compress pictures are Lossless JPEG, DICOM RLE, JPEG-LS and universal ones developed to standardize data representation but also to support compressing pictures: in the DICOM standard, the Deflate algorithm [16] is used in that fashion. It is also recommended to fully include such algorithms as JPEG2000, which already represent generally accepted standards, in the DICOM standard.

It is worth adding that when assessing the compression, measures of its effectiveness other than the compression rate defined and discussed above can be considered. Numerical measures of effectiveness include mainly: the compression percentage (CP) and the bit rate (BR).

Compression percentage (frequently used to assess the efficiency of text archiving tools) is defined as $CP = (1 - 1/CR)\ 100\%$, where the compression rate (CR) is the ratio of the number of bits of the original image representation to the number of bits of its compressed representation. Bit rate is the average number of bits of the compressed representation per one element of the source data sequence (in the case of image data, it is the average number of bits per pixel). The effectiveness (efficiency, capacity) of compression then means obtaining the highest possible CR and CP or the smallest possible BR.

CR and CP are relative measures, useful to e.g. evaluate how effective encoders are in archiving applications (their values can easily be translated into the amount of savings in storage media costs). The absolute value of BR characterizes the volume of output data from the encoder and is useful for transmission purposes (for example, it is easy to assess the required network speed in real time).

These analyses would be incomplete if we did not mention that the DICOM standard universally used in PACS systems defines, in addition to data compression methods, also the communication protocols used to transmit this data between remote institutions and the formats in which this data should be saved. As a result, the simple decision to choose and methodically apply the DICOM standard allows the user to forget the different details of medical image storage, processing and distribution, so this standard can be expected to be selected and applied more and more broadly.

3.8. Video sequence compression

In this book we focus mainly on analyzing, processing and recognizing single medical images or series of them produced by subsequent image examinations of some spatial fragment of a patient's body – e.g. a sequence of tomography slides which, when combined, are to present the 3D structure of the chest cavity or the brain. We do not, however, concentrate here on subjects related to video sequences generated by recording moving pictures.

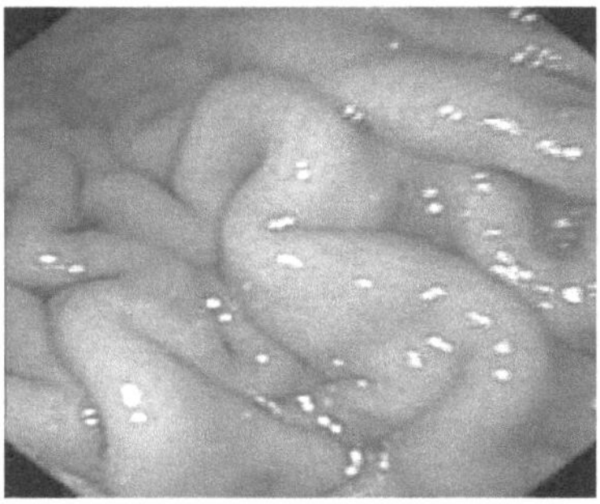

Fig. 3.9. Example of a gastroscopy image

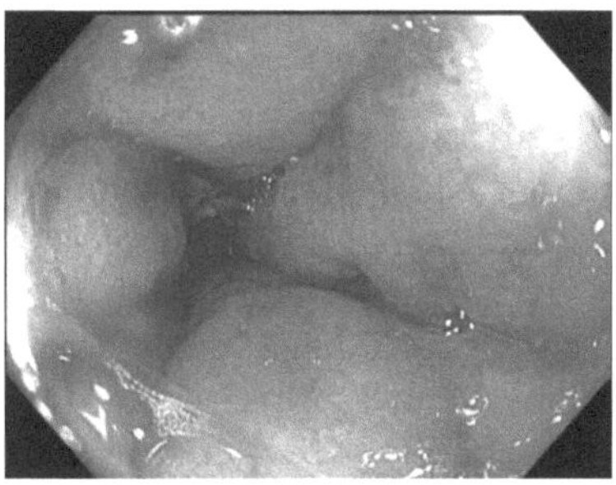

Fig. 3.10. Example of a colonoscopy image

However, without violating the above principle, it is worth hinting that current medical problems increasingly frequently make physicians use video recordings as the results of a specific examination of a patient. One situation in which a video recording can constitute an important part of medical documentation is any endoscopic examination. Depending on the organ examined, this may be a gastroscopy – Fig. 3.9 (of oesophagus and stomach, but sometimes even reaching the duodenum and then called duodenoscopy), rectoscopy or colonoscopy – Fig. 3.10 (aimed at observing the inside of the rectum, sigmoid and the large intestine), bronchoscopy – Fig. 3.11 (the observation of the inside of the trachea, bronchi and bronchioli) etc.

This list is by no means exhaustive, as the physicians are using increasingly better and more miniaturized endoscopes to reach more and more nooks and crannies of patients' bodies (examples include uroscopy – the internal observation of the urinary bladder and sometimes also ureters), and increasingly frequently view pictures from inside the human body while conducting surgical procedures by means of laparoscopy. During all these examinations, which provide very important information, but are hard and sometimes even dangerous for the patient, the recording of video images from the endoscope manipulated inside the body of the patient has become commonplace.

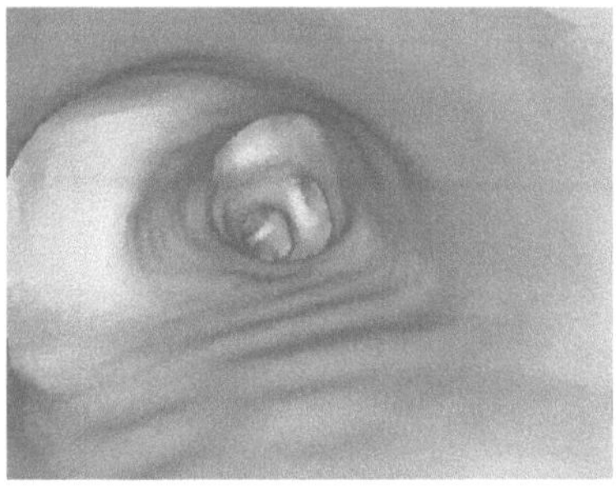

Fig. 3.11. Example of a bronchoscopy image

One feature of such recordings is that compared to the duration of the whole examination, the video sequence showing a diagnostically important picture is very short. For example, while the bronchoscope penetrates the bronchial tree, we can record thousands of images which show the speculum moving past healthy parts of the organ, and only a few will show signs of a tumor. Computer applications which would automatically review the recorded video sequences to detect and pinpoint (for the physician's assessment) only those suspicious images would help doctors a lot. However, to achieve this, we will have to collect digital recordings of the above video sequences and store them in patient documentation, but these recordings must be compressed (without compressing, they could not be stored in the memories of even the biggest computers).

Soon it will be necessary to consider video compression standards with a view to the needs brought about by their medical applications. However, we will not discuss this subject at greater length here. We just note that the popular MPEG-2 and the (more modern and better) H.264 standards seem to be the most promising video compression standards today.

3.9. The problem of assessing the quality of images subjected to compressing

Various methods of image compression have been compared in the previous subsection on the basis of the most obvious criterion, i.e. the compression rate. That is the best criterion for determining which methods are better and which worse if we are talking of **lossless** compression methods.

However, as we have mentioned in the previous parts of this chapter, lossy compression is increasingly frequently used to compact less sensitive (e.g. screening) medical images, based on the assumption that the information loss caused by the coding algorithm is really negligible, while the benefits provided by the much greater compression rate achievable by lossy compression and the much better compacting of the data stored or transmitted is very interesting.

However, there is a methodological problem in assessing the quality of medical images prior to and following their lossy compression. The problem is as follows: the measures of the degree of deformation caused by image compression (or some other way of its processing) are usually rather misleading.

The signal processing theory (most frequently of one-dimensional signals, like sounds) assumes that a measure of the deformation of these signals after lossy compression and decompression is the SSE (sum square errors): the total of squares of differences in the signal samples before and after the transformation assessed. This criterion was found to be useless for assessing the effect of image processing quite early on. If the values of the same pixels in the source and processed image are subtracted from one another and then the differences added up (after first squaring them so that positive and negative differences would not compensate each other), we get a numerical measurement of the deformation degree which is drastically inconsistent with the subjective judgments of people reviewing these images. Frequently, images with relatively low SSEs are visually found to be significantly different, while it is very easy to show transformations which actually do not distort the image at a all, but generate very high SSE values. One such transformation is a tiny shift of image contents, without changing them at all. To an observer, the shifted image looks exactly the same as the original but the SSEs of these two images are very different, because the relevant points do not coincide, so almost every pixel is classified as erroneous.

In order to avoid such paradoxes, other measures of the similarity (or difference) between compared images are looked for. Currently, the greatest hopes rest on a measure called structural similarity (SSIM), described in [63]. However, a detailed discussion of this measure exceeds the scope of this chapter.

4. Preprocessing medical images and their overall enhancement

This chapter briefly discusses the main stages of image preprocessing. The introduction to this book mentioned that the preprocessing of medical image is subject to certain restrictions and is generally more complex than the processing of other image types [26, 52]. This is why, of the many different techniques and methods for image filtering, we have decided to discuss here only selected ones, most frequently applied to medical images and which have been proven to be suitable for that purpose in numerous practical cases. Their operation will be illustrated with examples of simple procedures aimed at improving the quality of imaging and allowing significant information to be generated for its use at the stages of image interpretation.

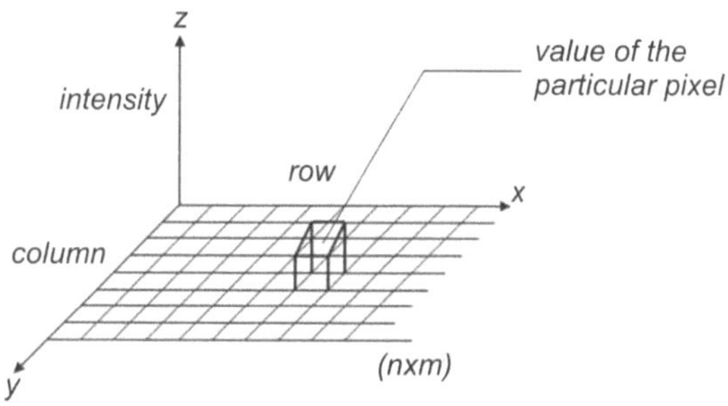

Fig. 4.1. Interpreting an image as a 2D function

When considering various filtering methods for an image, it is good to refer to its interpretation as a function with two variables (Fig. 4.1). This interpretation is presented in Fig. 4.2 in an even more illustrative way.

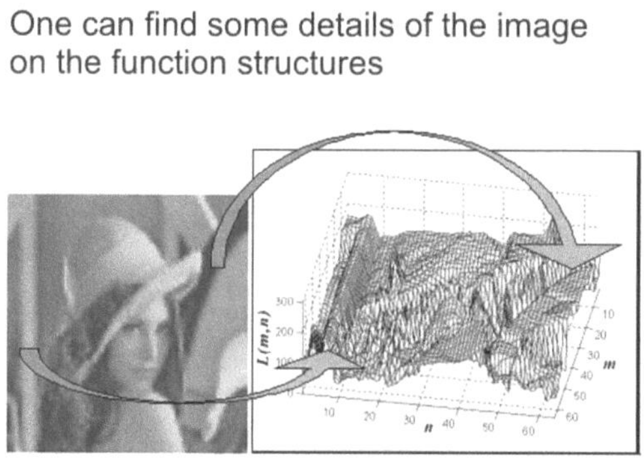

Fig. 4.2. Relationships between image elements and details of a 2D function used to represent it in a computer processing system

M.R. Ogiela and R. Tadeusiewicz: *Preprocessing medical images and their overall enhancement,* Studies in Computational Intelligence (SCI) **84**, 65–97 (2007)
www.springerlink.com

4.1. One point based transformations

The simplest class of computer image processing methods contains **single-point operations,** which are image processing methods based on the principle of generating one pixel of the output image on the basis of a single pixel of the input (original) image. It is easy to see that this principle of operation excludes from the start the possibility of obtaining any new (additional) information as a result of completing the planned actions, Fig. 4.3. On the contrary, selected operations of this group may lead to some information being **lost** (if pixels of **various** values in the original image receive **identical** values after processing). So from the point of view of the subsequent, objective (computer performed) stages of processing, analyzing, recognizing and even automatically understanding images, these operations yield no result.

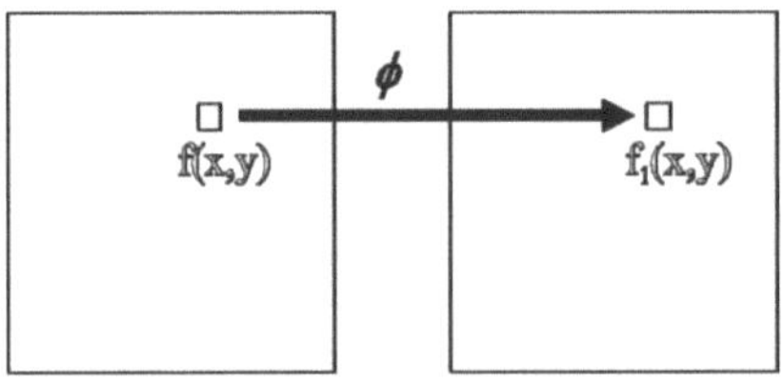

$$f_1(x,y) = \phi[f(x,y)]$$

Fig. 4.3. A diagram of a single-point operation

However, in the realm of medical images, the objective (information theory related) characteristics of these images are really of only secondary importance. What is of key importance is the **subjective** information which the image presents to the physician and to what extent this subjective information can contribute to improving his/her work, in particular to making correct diagnostic decisions. And it is here that single-point operations are very useful, as by selecting the right grey levels (and sometimes also artificial colors), we can make what is recorded in the picture more visible. An example of this is given in Fig. 4.4.

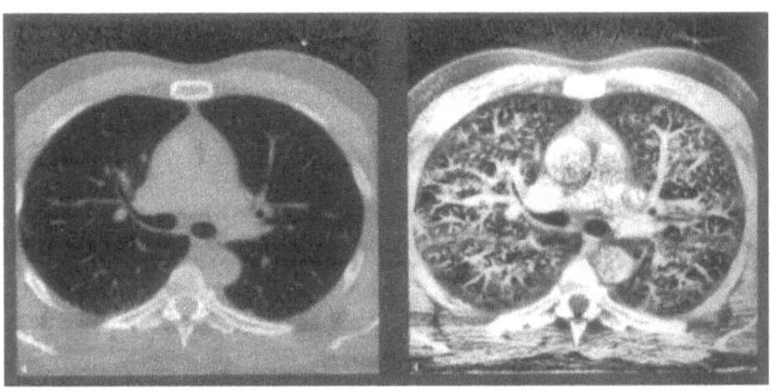

Fig. 4.4. A single-point transformation of an image can make it more legible to the human eye, even though it actually causes some information loss

In this picture, the left hand side tomogram has been presented the way it looks after recording (the different levels of X-ray absorption by tissues correspond to various grey levels). Due to the absorption of a very broad range between the highest and the lowest absorption values, small differences are almost invisible. However, on the right hand side, the same image is shown without presenting the whole X-ray absorption scale, but only selecting a certain range of these values, with the values from that range shown as different grey levels. Consequently, the right hand side image in Fig. 4.4 contains a great deal less information than the one on the left, but it is more legible to humans and therefore easier to translate into the correct diagnosis.

By combining single point transformations with selected image analysis techniques (in particular with segmentation techniques discussed in the following chapter), we can cause only the fragment of the image containing the necessary information to be selected for analyzing (visually or algorithmically), while the remaining anatomical details will be removed from the image – Fig. 4.5. This results in a major loss of abundant information, so if the image is to be assessed visually by a doctor, we usually do not apply such radical methods. However, if automatic methods of image recognition or understanding are to be applied, this approach can be very useful to simplify the job to be performed by the classification algorithm.

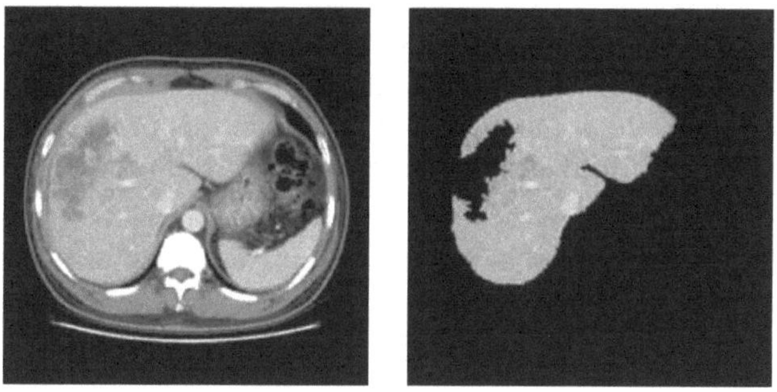

Fig. 4.5. Single-point transformations allow just the outline of the organ being assessed to be extracted from the entire X-ray photograph

An undisputed advantage of single-point transformations is the speed at which they can be completed. Even if the Φ function shown in Fig. 4.1 is very complex, its value has to be calculated only as many times as there are pixels in the image. Today's computing technology means that this takes fractions of a second even for images that contain more than ten million pixels. In this respect, context transformations described in the following chapter are less efficient.

Literature describes a very broad range of single-point image transformations, and on top of them, one can use transformations in which the Φ function is freely set by the user as a graphic relationship between the brightness of pixels in the source image (on the horizontal axis) and the brightness of pixels in the output image (on the vertical axis), Fig. 4.6. Such freely set transformations are usually achieved using the technique of look-up-tables.

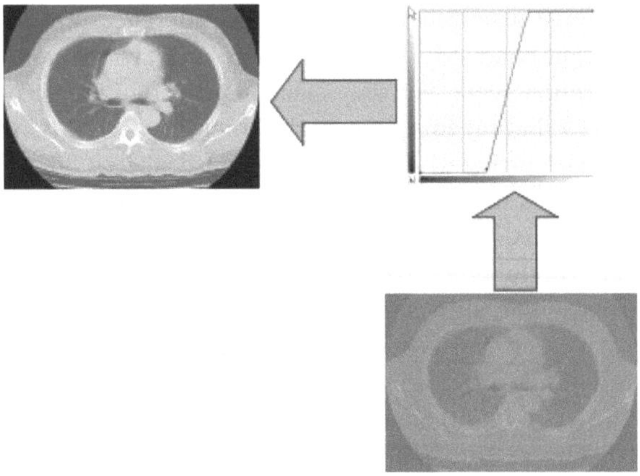

Fig. 4.6. Making a single-point transformation set by a graphically displayed function

However, it is not always easy to imagine what transformation will enhance the desirable characteristics of the image, so there is a need to adopt some standard solution for this problem. A standard that works relatively well is the histogram equalization technique. Its starting point is to determine the histogram of the image. That, as we know, is the result of calculating how many instances of pixels of a specific brightness the picture has. The horizontal axis of the histogram shows grey levels, and the vertical axis represents the number of pixels of that grey level (Fig. 4.7).

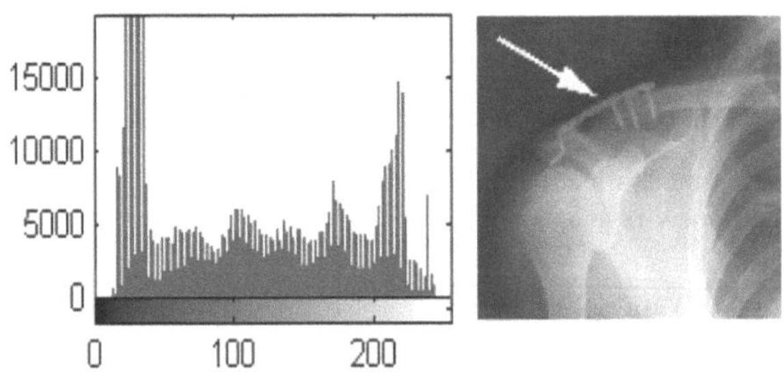

Fig. 4.7. An example histogram of a medical image

The histogram provides a wealth of valuable information about the image (Fig. 4.8) and also suggests what transformation should be applied to the image so that what is visible in it would become even better and more clearly visible. The principle is simple: the taller the bar, the more distant it should be from other bars.

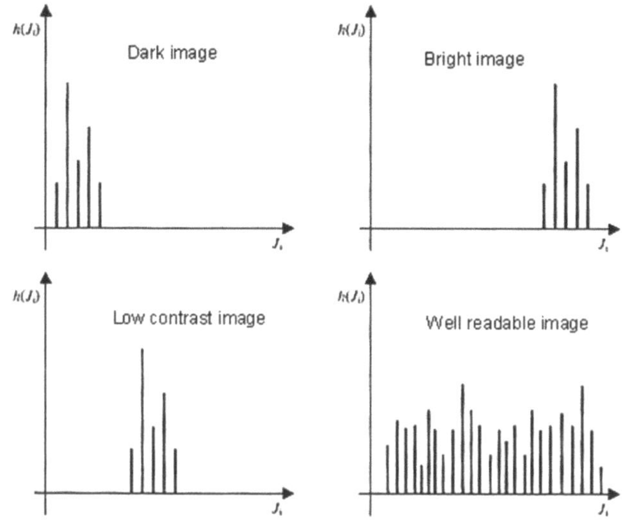

Fig. 4.8. Examples of histograms of incorrect and correct images

Fig. 4.9 shows how this method works, and Fig. 4.10 presents an example of using histogram equalization to obtain a correct medical diagnosis.

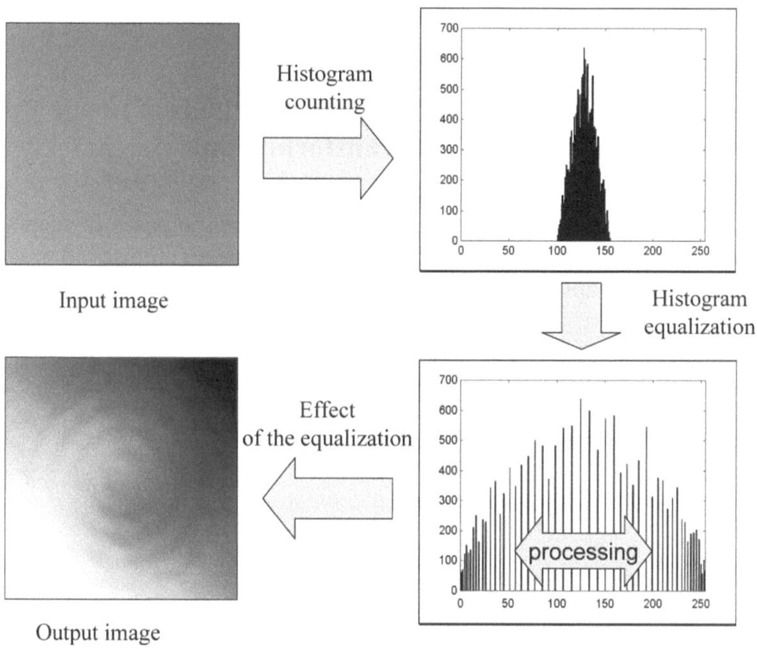

Fig. 4.9. A histogram equalization procedure and its result

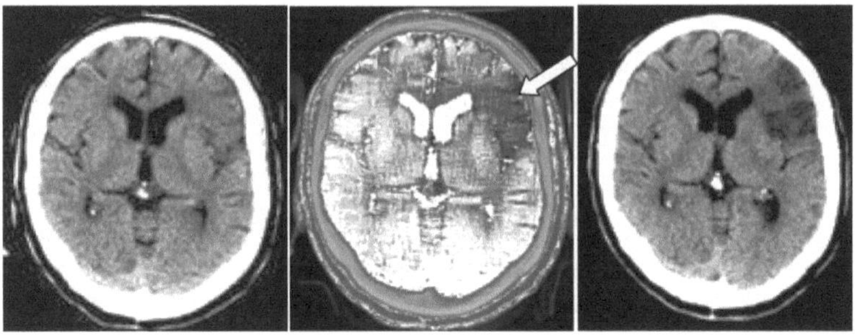

A B C

Fig. 4.10. Results of histogram equalization and their impact on the diagnosis. Described in the text

Fig. 4.10 A shows a CT of the brain **directly** after an injury which caused an ischemia of the right hemisphere. Almost nothing is visible in the original image! Fig. 4.10 B shows the same tomogram after histogram equalization. The ischemia of the right hemisphere has become visible and enables an early diagnosis to be made, which is necessary for the correct treatment. The correctness of the image generated by the computer and shown in Fig. 4.10 B is confirmed by a CT scan made 4 days later, shown in Fig. 4.10 C. In this image, the ischemia is clearly visible without any image processing, but at this stage, treatment would have been late and unsuccessful.

4.2. Subtractive angiography and other methods of image enrichment using multi-image transformations

Single point operations are sometimes used for medical purposes in such a way that single pixels of several (most often two) source images are used to produce a single pixel of the output image: Fig. 4.11.

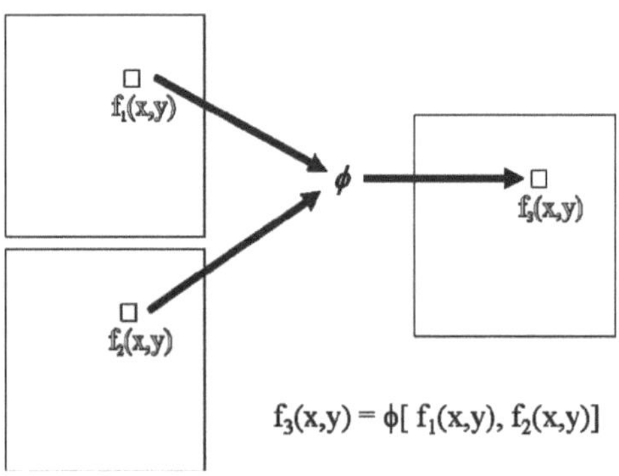

Fig. 4.11. A diagram of generating the output image by a single-point, two-argument operation

The most popular way of using this image operation model is to **subtract** two images from each other to disclose changes which took place between the recording of the first and of the second image. As image subtraction is used, this group of imaging techniques is frequently referred to as subtraction methods.

The most frequent reason why the aforementioned change takes place between the recording time of the first and the second image which are to be subtracted is the administering of a contrast medium, whose presence in the examined organ makes it visible in the image, e.g. in an X-ray or a CT scan. This begs the following question: if the appropriate structures become visible in an X-ray after the contrast is administered, why perform any other operations, e.g. a subtraction?

The reason is that an X-ray of an organ containing contrast is not always easy to view. This is because in such a picture, apart from the anatomical structures of interest, which are filled with the contrast (but still not always easily visible), there are also images of other structures (e.g. fragments of the skeleton, which are always very obvious in X-ray photographs), which images make the doctor's analysis of significant details difficult. But if we subtract the X-ray photograph taken without the contrast from that in which the specific structure has already filled with contrast, the differential image is much easier to interpret: Fig. 4.12.

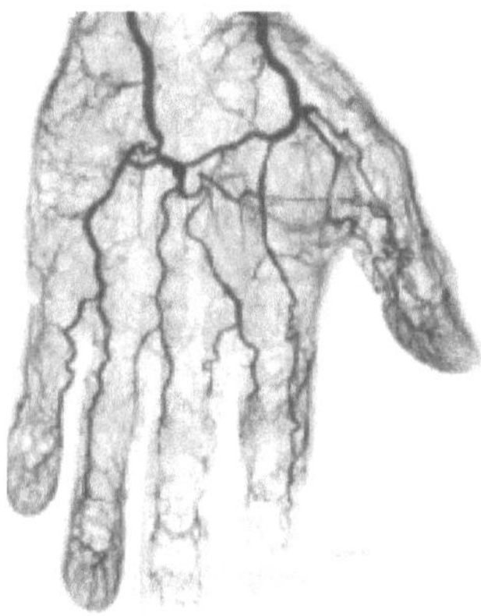

Fig. 4.12. The result of subtracting the image of a hand with contrast administered from that containing no contrast. It is mainly the contrast-filled blood vessels that are visible

The organs easiest to fill with contrast media are various kinds of vessels (including blood vessels, see Fig. 4.12, but also other vessels, like urethers or the pancreatic duct in the case of the ERCP examination), so the technique for enhancing the image using subtractive methods is frequently referred to as **angiography.**

Digital Subtraction Angiography (DSA) is a technique used to improve the contrast of soft tissue images shown in X-ray pictures. In practice, bone tissues images generally contrast well with the background, while in the case of soft tissues, the contrast is generally poor, making them difficult to assess.

This problem also applies to the visualization of blood vessels, which is important when assessing the degree of arteriosclerotic lesions, detecting aneurysms, hemorrhages and narrowings of the opening of blood vessels.

In simple terms, the DSA consists in taking an X-ray photograph of the examined part of the patient's body and intravenously administering a contrast medium to that patient after that photograph has been taken. The next stage is to take another photograph, which clearly shows blood vessels containing the contrast medium. Once we have both images, we subtract them from each other, and obtain an image showing only the vessels set out by the contrast medium. The image is used to make the diagnosis. As the subtraction means deducting the information contained in a given image point from the information contained in the same point of the other image, it is crucial that both photographs show exactly the same area of the patient's body. If these areas are shifted, artifacts may appear, and will interfere with or completely prohibit further image analysis.

Subtractive angiography generates images of better contrast and quality than those produced by classical angiography. It also requires much less contrast medium.

Subtractive angiography can also be used in cases where a whole sequence of images acquired during one procedure for distinguishing vessel morphology (e.g. a coronarography examination of coronary arteries) is used to distinguish the structure searched for (the contrasted vessel). This type of filtering makes it possible to isolate the structure to be found on the basis of local changes in contrasts occurring during the transition from one image of the sequence to the next. This is possible, as anatomic structures which are not shifted or contrasted while the sequence of such images is recorded generate information with the temporary frequency of 0 Hz. On the contrary, small movements caused by the patient's breathing during the acquisition of a sequence of images may generate information with a frequency below the range resulting from the heart action, i.e. 1 Hz – 2 Hz. Frequency filters eliminate all frequency components below 1 Hz.

Generally, this method is used to filter as follows. Let I_j be the sequence of j images: for any j moment, we can generate an M_j filtration map by adding up several images obtained so far, e.g.:

$$M_j = I_{j-1} + I_{j-2} + \ldots + I_{j-n}$$

where:

$n \times \delta t$ – time interval of acquiring n images;

δt – the time between acquiring two subsequent images (1/30 s is the standard).

Temporal frequencies appearing below $1/(n \times \delta t)$ are eliminated by subtracting M_j from the last image in the I_j sequence.

Images binarized in the above way are then subjected to an edge smoothing procedure, e.g. the averaging and median filtering of the image, which eliminates all irregularities present on the outer side of edges of the organs examined. Using the generally accepted image algebra notation, both filtering operations can be represented by the following formulas.

1. Averaging filter [48]

$$b(y) = 1/n \Sigma_{x \in N(y)} a(x), \ for \ \forall y \in a$$

where:
a – original input image;
b – output image obtained by averaging the neighborhood of subsequent points;
$a(x)$ – the grey level of a point with the x coordinate (where $x \in Z^2$) in the input image;
$b(y)$ – the grey level of a point with the y coordinate in the output image;
n – the number of points belonging to the neighborhood $N(y)$ of the y image.

2. Median filter [48]

$$b(y)=med\{a(x), x \in N(y)\} \ for \ \forall y \in a$$

where *med* is a function determining the median value for the neighborhood of point $a(x)$.

Such transformations change the contents of the image or the geometry of objects visible in it, at the same time help to eliminate various types of distortions or noise, and enhance useful information. Median filtering is very effective in eliminating all local noise. It also does not introduce any new values, so the output image does not require any additional scaling, neither does that filtering cause any blurring of edges of individual objects visible in the filtered image.

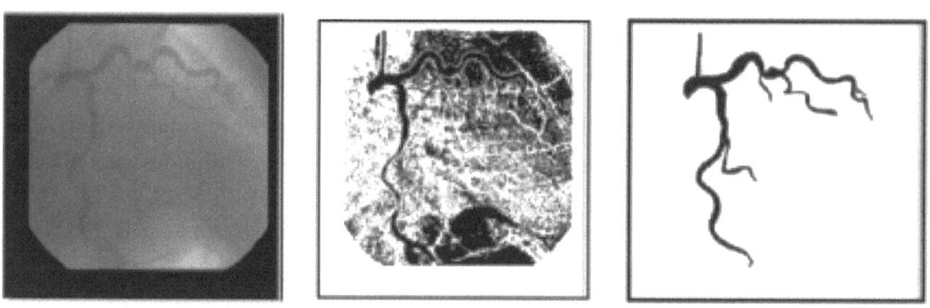

A B C

Fig. 4.13. An image of coronary arteries: **A** – with contrast medium administered, **B** – a more contrasting image obtained by histogram equalization, **C** – an image obtained by angiography

In conditions which support its good application, angiography yields a much better imaging of structures material for diagnoses than any other imaging method (compare Fig. 4.13 B and C, obtained from the same image shown in Fig. 4.13 A).

4.3. Simple low pass and high pass filtering of images

4.3.1. General definition

Low pass, morphological, gradient and other high pass filters belong to contextual operations. Nowadays, there are many operations performed on images, whose joint characteristic is that calculations of **many** points of the source image are necessary to determine the value of one point of the output image. A contextual operation, which refers to a specific pixel in the output image, consists of determining the value of a function whose main arguments are the value of the source image pixel which has the same position as the pixel being calculated, and the values of pixels surrounding it. The calculated value of the above function is then substituted as the new value of the pixel in question. Usually, the surrounding area taken into account when executing contextual operations consists of points surrounding the point being processed (grey points in Fig. 4.14). Those points delineate the so-called direct neighborhood (grey points in Fig. 4.14) or the indirect neighborhood (white points in Fig. 4.14). Computer analysis may make use of the so-called neighborhood schemes (called masks) which define only direct neighbors or masks containing both direct and indirect neighbors.

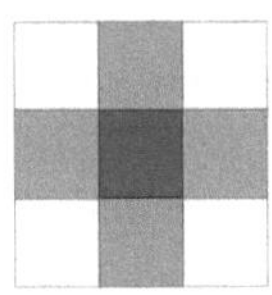

Fig. 4.14. The structure of point surroundings during contextual filtering

As contextual operations like filtering make use of pixels surrounding the pixel being processed, they may turn out to be impossible in the case of pixels located at the limits of the image, as there are no arguments. Such a situation is illustrated in Figure 4.15, where the neighborhood for points on the image edge requires going beyond the image area.

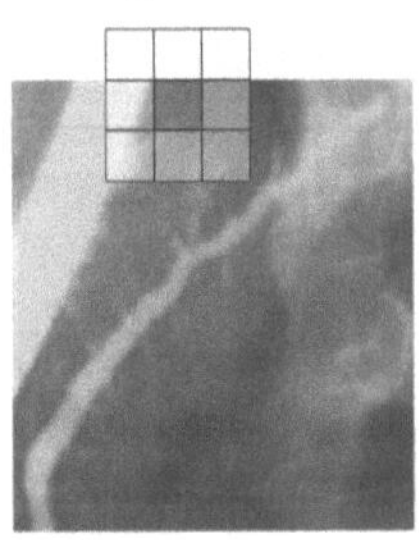

Fig. 4.15. An example where contextual filtering cannot be conducted for points on the edges of the image (the enlarged area corresponding to the filtration mask can be seen)

Regardless of this limitation, image filtering operations are very frequently used to process and analyze the image. Unlike point operations, they significantly change image contents, including the geometry of objects visible in it. They can successfully eliminate some undesirable components, such as interference or noise, and also extract certain information invisible in the original image.

Filters are divided into linear and non-linear. A filter is classified as linear if the φ function that it executes meets two linearity conditions:

- it is additive $\varphi(f+g)=\varphi(f)+\varphi(g)$
- and it is uniform $\varphi(\lambda f)=\lambda\varphi(f), \lambda \in \Re$

where: φ – function executed by the filter, f, g – images subjected to filtering

Linear filters most frequently used in practice include those which additionally meet the condition of constancy in relation to a shift:

$$\varphi(f_{\vec{h}})=\left[\varphi(f)\right]_{\vec{h}}\text{, where } h \text{ is the shift vector}$$

If this condition is fulfilled, every point of the image subjected to the operation of the filter will be transformed in the same way.

Filters used in linear image filtration usually operate in accordance with the convolution rule. This rule consists in executing the following operation for every image point determined by the x and y coordinates:

$$f'(x,y)=\sum_{(i,j)\in M} f(x+i,y+j)\cdot W_{i,j}$$

In this formula, $f(x,y)$ denotes the value of the source image pixel (c.f. Fig. 4.16) with the coordinates of x and y, whereas $f'(x,y)$ is an auxiliary value which, after normalization (see below) will constitute the value of the corresponding output image pixel. The ancillary variables i and j run across the inside of an assumed area M, which constitutes the neighborhood of point (x,y) illustratively shown in Fig. 4.14, and is also known as the convolution window. It is worth noting that i and j can take both positive and negative values, as the M neighborhood is usually symmetrical in relation to point (x,y).

It is worth noting that pixel values defined specifically as the grey levels of specific points in the image must be integers from a strictly defined range of values (usually [0, 255] due to the single-byte representations of pixels). However, the result of calculations defined by the above formula determining the value of $f'(x,y)$ obviously need not meet those conditions. For example, if a low pass filtering is applied, all $W_{i,j}$ coefficients will be positive integers of various values, but in that case the maximum value that can be taken by $f'(x,y)$ may be significantly greater than the limit of 255. It gets even worse in high pass filtering, as then $W_{i,j}$ coefficients are either positive and negative integers, so the output value of $f'(x,y)$ may be either positive or negative. Consequently, in both cases the calculated value of $f'(x,y)$ must be adjusted before it is substituted as the value of the output image pixel, whereas the adjustment formula may be defined in various ways. However, as the above adjustment is really just a certain simple result scaling (usually calculated as a look-up table), we will not be discussing it in detail here.

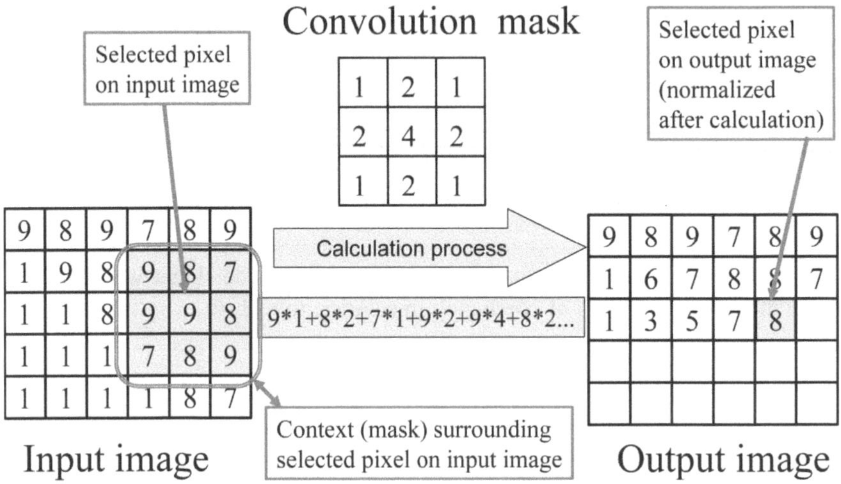

Fig. 4.16. Illustration of the operation of a contextual transformation

The type of a transformation performed on the image as a result of the execution of the operator described above depends on the value of $W_{i,j}$ coefficients defined by the convolution matrix (mask) adopted. An example structure of such a mask for a convolution window with the dimensions of 3 × 3 (i.e. of the structure shown in Fig.4.14) is presented below:

W[1,1]	W[1,0]	W[1,-1]
W[0,1]	W[o,o]	W[O,-1]
W[-1,1]	W[-1,0]	W[-1,-1]

Having defined the values of the $W_{i,j}$ coefficients, we get a tool which can be specifically considered as a linear filter modifying the entire image being processed.

Linear filters are divided into low pass and high pass filters. These names refer to notions known from filtering simple one-dimensional signals (e.g. the speech signal) where low pass filtration means that signal components of low frequencies pass through the filter, while high frequency components (usually noise) are stopped by the filter. High pass filtration, on the other hand, means that high frequency components pass through the filter (this amplifies moments in which the signal changes rapidly and suddenly).

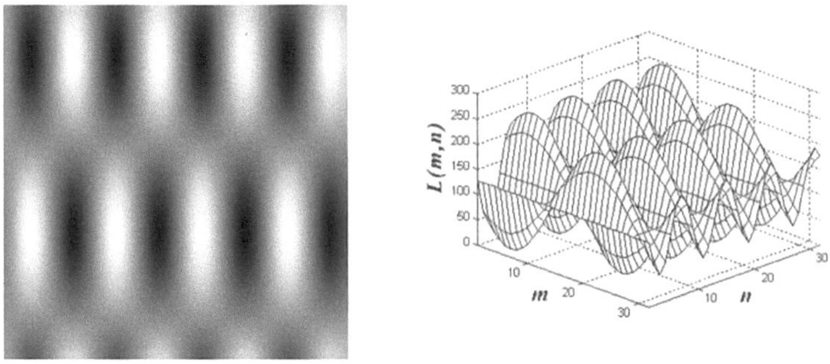

A B

Fig. 4.17. An artificial image in which the brightness changes with a greater frequency along the horizontal axis and with a lower frequency along the vertical axis. A – an image represented using grey levels, B – an image represented by a graph of a function with two variables

In the case of images, which are two-dimensional signals (see Fig. 4.1), the notion of frequency gets complicated, as the variability observed in the image along one axis may be different from the variability along the other axis. This is illustrated by Fig. 4.17, an artificially generated image with a high frequency of changes along the horizontal axis and a low frequency of changes along the vertical one (this is visible more precisely in Fig. 4.17 B, where that artificial image is presented as a function of two variables whose x and y coordinates are the respective coordinates of pixels in the image, while the function values (vertical components in the graph) correspond to the brightness of particular image points). A review of the presented image shows that just saying that we are dealing with a high or a low frequency is not sufficient for an image. To provide complete information, we should also indicate whether we are talking of a high or a low frequency and along which direction the frequency of changes is as described.

This circumstance is less important for low pass filters, whose directional action is usually mitigated by adopting a set of $W_{i,j}$ coefficients characterized by central symmetry, while for high pass filters, the directional action of the filter is intentionally used to obtain specific special effects in the processed image.

4.3.2. Low pass filters

If the convolution mask is filled with only positive values of $W_{i,j}$ coefficients, it gives us a low pass filter. The most popular use of low pass filters is to eliminate interference from images. Usually, a simple averaging filter is used for this purpose, whose mask is shown in Fig. 4.18.

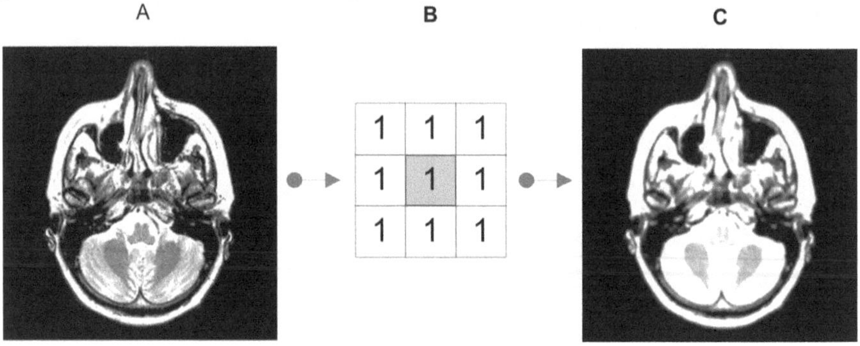

Fig. 4.18. A head CT scan subjected to averaging filtering. A) The original image before filtering, B) The averaging filter mask, C) The image after filtering through a low pass filter

It is easy to see in the drawing (Fig. 4.18) that this filter removes or significantly reduces small interferences of the image and smoothes some edges. Small changes of brightness in any given area are also mitigated. Unfortunately, this filter also yields some undesirable effects, such as the blurred contours of anatomic structures visible in the image and making their shapes more difficult to recognize.

To mitigate the negative effects of such averaging filtering, sometimes filters with an amplified central point (or also its direct neighborhood) of the mask are used, which means that the original value of the pixel has a greater impact on its value in the output image after filtering. Examples of such filters and the results of their application are presented in Fig. 4.19 and 4.20.

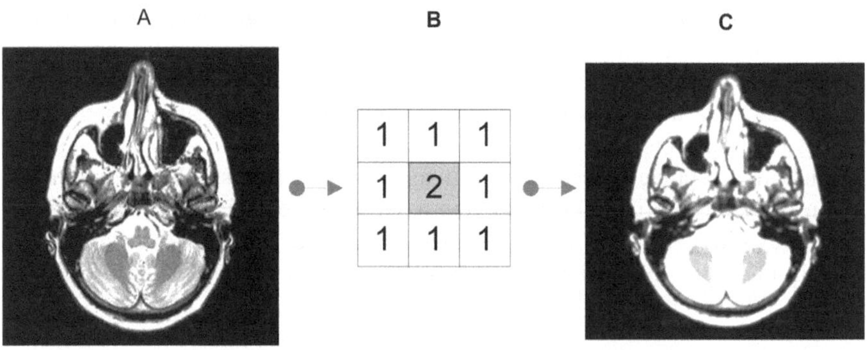

Fig. 4.19. A head CT scan subjected to averaging filtering with an amplified central point of the filtration mask. A) The original image prior to filtering, B) The mask of the averaging filter, C) The image after filtering through a low pass filter

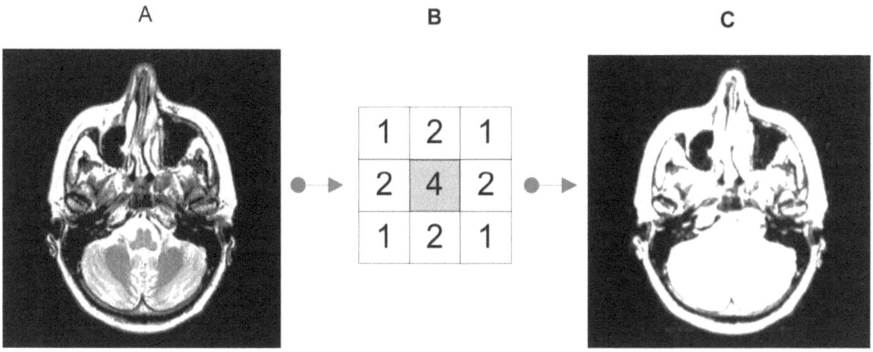

Fig. 4.20. A head CT scan subjected to averaging filtering with an even more amplified central point and its direct neighborhood. A) The original image prior to filtering, B) The mask of the averaging filter, C) The image after filtering through a low pass filter

Sometimes filters are used that feature a mask which is not amplified in the centre, but, on the contrary, weakens the influence of that point on the final filtering result. The effects of this operation can be observed in Fig. 4.21.

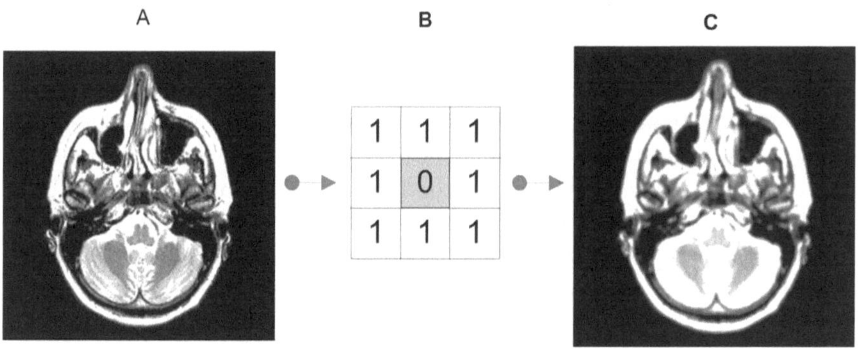

Fig. 4.21. A head CT scan subjected to averaging filtering with a weakened central point of the filtering mask. A) The original image prior to filtering, B) The mask of the averaging filter, C) The image after filtering without amplification in the centre

The presented examples show that low pass filters may feature different definitions of the function for transferring information from the input to the output image, but they have one thing in common: while removing interferences from the image, they also undesirably contribute to reducing the contrast of images and may therefore eliminate some material information about the edges or the texture of selected areas or structures. Consequently, such filters are dedicated to specific jobs of analyzing one type of imaging and the results of their application are usually combined with procedures that compensate image blurring.

4.3.3. High pass filters

Another group of filters are high pass filters used to isolate elements responsible for rapid brightness changes, e.g. contours and edges, from the image. In general, such operations are said to enhance edges of objects in the image. We can say that high pass filters act by signal differentiation. The simplest example of such a filter is the Roberts gradient. The filter mask and the result of filter application are presented in Fig. 4.22.

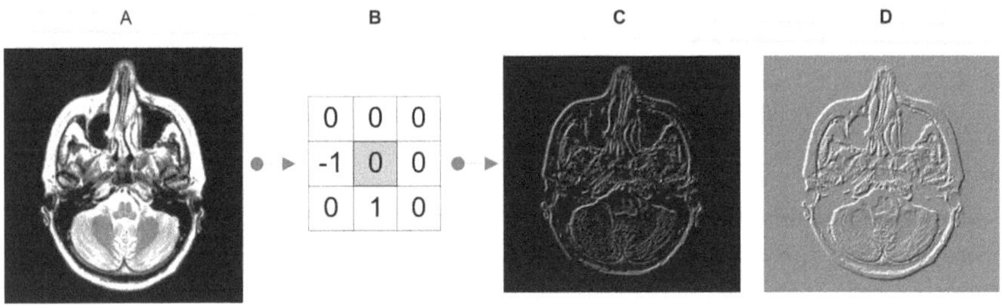

Fig. 4.22. A head CT scan subjected to focusing filtration with a Roberts filter. A) The original image prior to filtering, B) The Roberts gradient mask, C) The skull CT image after filtering with the Roberts filter, D) The image after filtering with Roberts filter an scaling

The effects of applying such a gradient are shown in Fig. 4.22. We can see that the distinguished directions of edges have been enhanced, but as the filter mask contains positive and negative coefficients, the output image may contain pixels with positive or negative values which clearly do not match the set of values defined as the allowed (and interpreted) grey levels of analyzed images. Consequently, to obtain a correct image, absolute values of pixels must be used, or the image must be scaled (Fig. 4.22.D). Unfortunately, scaling makes the background brighter, positive pixels very dark, and negative pixels brighter than the background.

The Roberts gradient, as one can see in Fig. 4.22, is directional and enhances lines of a certain orientation, depending on the mask used. For directions perpendicular to those currently considered, the mask is defined in the same way but as a mirror reflection of a value in relation to the centre column.

This type of direction or corner-detecting gradients [47] is used in medical image analysis to detect and describe the edges of the structures analyzed. Figure 4.23 shows an example set of masks for edge-detection filters running in specific directions (the location of a specific mask in the diagram shows what directional structures are detected by this mask).

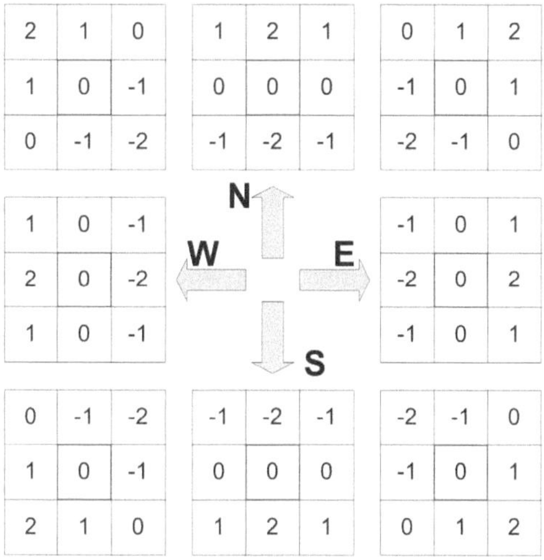

Fig. 4.23. A set of masks generating gradients of images of various directions

The effects of applying masks shown in Fig. 4.23 are presented in Fig. 4.24. Individual parts of this figure, occupied by the relevant masks in Fig. 4.23, show the effects of using these masks. These effects are demonstrated using not a medical image, but a picture of a sailboat, as the effects of gradient operations are easier to detect on a simpler picture (of the sailboat).

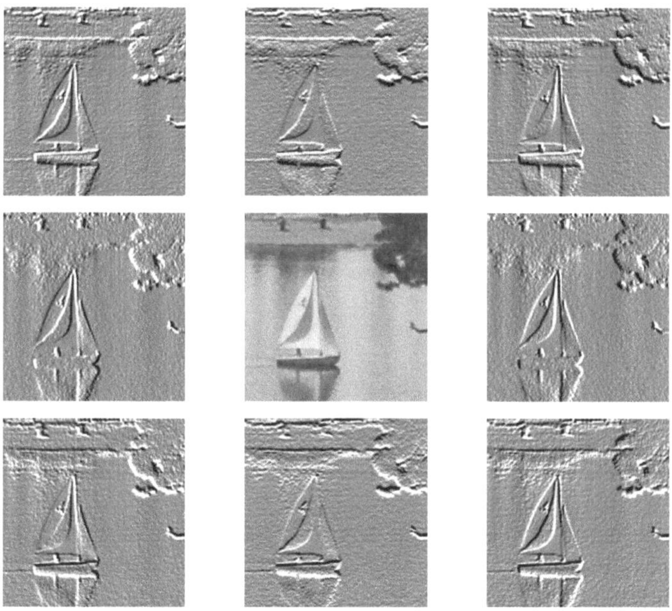

Fig. 4.24. Effects of using gradients whose masks are shown in Fig. 23. The original image being processed is situated in the middle of the frame

The above high pass filters calculate (with better or worse results) the **first derivatives** of an image signal, which allows the contours of objects visible in the image to be determined, but only as long as these are mainly the contours and edges running in a specific, determined direction. However, we would often like to detect all contours and edges in the image, regardless of the direction in which they run. For such edge detection, it is best to use an operator which determines (approximately, of course) the value of the **second derivative** of the image. The appropriate operator is created (inter alia) when one of the convolution masks shows in Fig. 4.25 is used.

0	-1	0
-1	4	-1
0	-1	0

-1	-1	-1
-1	8	-1
-1	-1	-1

-1	-2	-1
-2	4	-2
-1	-2	-1

0	-1	0
-1	5	-1
0	-1	0

-1	-1	-1
-1	9	-1
-1	-1	-1

-1	-2	-1
-2	5	-2
-1	-2	-1

Fig. 4.25. Examples of edge detection filter masks – Laplacians

Determining the edges allows one to concentrate on the key features of the medical image examined: for example in an image of heart cavities it allows the cavity and atrium volume as well as the wall thickness to be determined – Fig. 4.26.

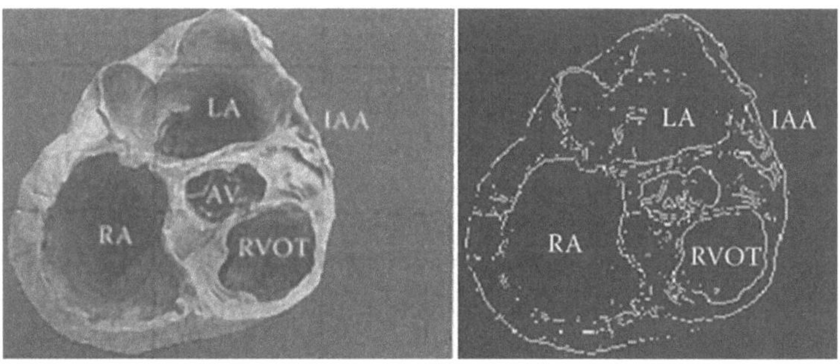

Fig. 4.26. Contour isolation as a technique that helps to analyze a medical image (source Internet)

In conclusion, it can be said that depending on the type of filtering applied, the same medical image may greatly change in appearance, which allows it to be analyzed in different ways and helps to isolate, or conversely hide certain of its characteristics. This is shown in a general way in Fig. 4.27.

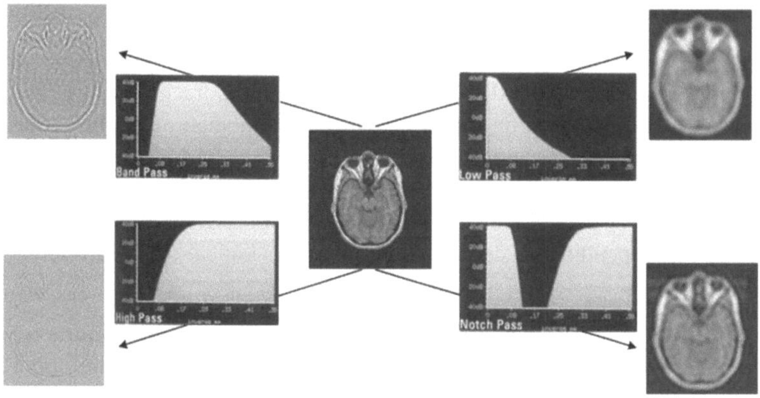

Fig. 4.27. The same medical image subjected to different filtering

4.4. Nonlinear filtering and mathematical morphology algorithms for medical image cleaning and improvement

Nonlinear filters are those that use various nonlinear transformations of signals and which support more complicated image filtering than that done with linear filters. One of the simplest methods of nonlinear image transformation is to apply the so-called combined filters. They act by applying two gradients along directions perpendicular to one another and then nonlinearly combining the outputs (images) obtained by using these gradients. This filter generates results better than linear filtration, which, in the case of enhancing contours in the image, can yield a very clear image with enhanced contours regardless of the direction in which they run: Fig. 4.28.

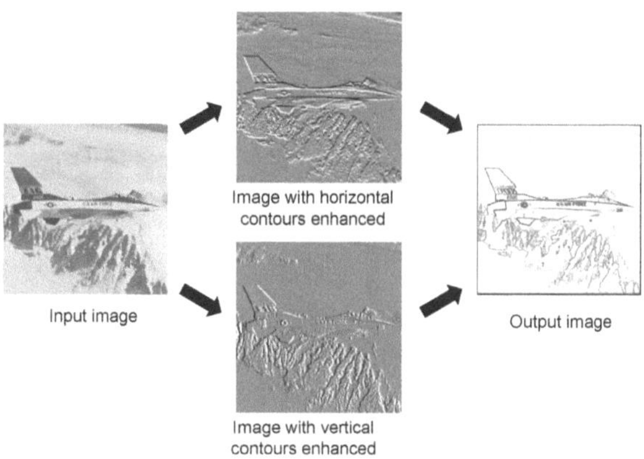

Fig. 4.28. The effect of a combined filter

Nonlinear filters are used in medical practice to obtain the following effects:

- To dampen noise and other distortions occurring in the image. In this case, the filter usually works based on the principles of the median of the brightness of points surrounding the processed pixel;
- Amplifying certain elements of the image which are consistent with a pattern set by a defined structural element or neighborhood. A given point is amplified or dampened depending on certain conditions, e.g. logical ones, fulfilled by its surroundings.

One example of a nonlinear filter is a median filter which supports a very radical removal of minor interferences appearing in the image. The operating principle of a median filter is as follows:

For the processed point of the output image, the median filter selects the middle (median) value of the sorted values of that point and its surroundings in the source image.

A median filter is classified among filters of a very radical action, as even extreme values of disturbed pixels which are much different from the average for a given region of the image have no impact on the value obtained on the output of the filter. An example of the operation of a median filter is shown in Fig. 4.29.

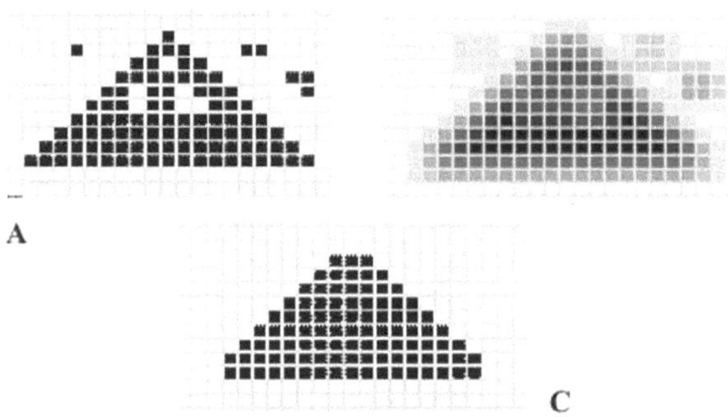

Fig. 4.29. An example of the operation of a median filter compared to the operation of a linear filter for convolution filtering. A – A fragment of disturbed image, B – The same image fragment after filtering with a convolution filter, C – The same fragment of the image after median filtering

When you look at Fig. 4.29, note the following details. Convolution filtering has not cleaned up the image precisely: in the place where the interferences originally occurred (black spots on a white background or the other way around), traces of these interferences are left after filtering in the form of fuzzy grey spots on a white background and (less visible) fuzzy grey spots on a black background. In addition, we can see how the convolution filter mutilated object edges, which used to be sharp in the original. The median filter has left no trace of the interferences removed, both in the case of removing the dark spots on a white background and of the reverse polarization. The image also bears out the claim that the main advantage of median filtering is that it usually does not reduce the sharpness of object edges found in the image being filtered: this can also be observed in Fig. 4.29. It is also worth noting that this filtering does not introduce new values into the image, so it is not necessary to additionally scale signal amplitudes allocated to particular pixels after the filtering is completed.

The drawbacks of the median may include the unavoidable erosion of particularly small fragments of the image, which can be observed in Fig. 4.29 in the corners of the triangle shown in it. This erosion will apply to all minor details of the image, particularly those on the edges of objects, which the median filter treats as interferences. Another drawback of the median technique is the time-consuming nature of this filtering process, as the lengthy sorting operation has to be conducted many times (in each position of the window moved around in the image). However, with today's fast computers, the delay caused by median filtering in the image processing process is negligible, particularly for a neighborhood of 3×3. However, we frequently need the image prepro sor to run faster, and then all such operations are implemented in hardware arrays (usually FPGA reprogrammable arrays) which allow the image to be processed immediately, that is within a time shorter than that needed to acquire that image.

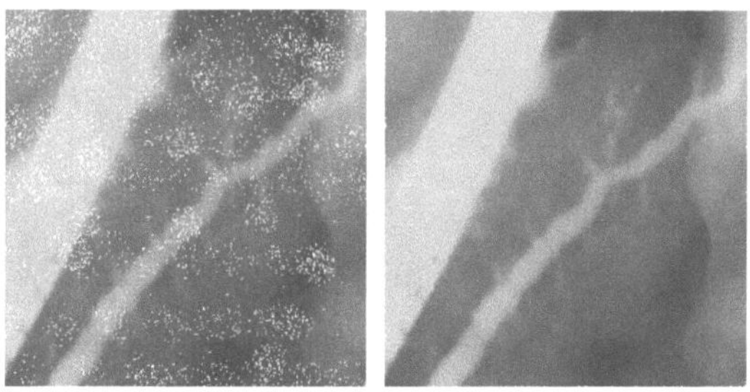

Fig. 4.30. The effect of denoising using median filtering. A) A noisy ERCP image, B) The image after median filtering with a 3x3 mask

Median filtering alone is most frequently used to eliminate noise from an image. Fig. 4.30 shows examples of median operation during the elimination of noise from a grey scale image.

A special class of nonlinear image transformations that help obtain images whose characteristics are more suitable for interpreting during the process of diagnostic decision making are **morphology transformations.** The basic notion for morphological transformations is the ***structuring element of the image.*** This is a certain fragment of the image (a specific subset of elements) with a single point – the central point – distinguished. The most popular structuring element is a unit radius circle, whereas due to the discrete nature of the raster building the medical image, the notion of a "circle" has to be modified appropriately (Fig. 4.31).

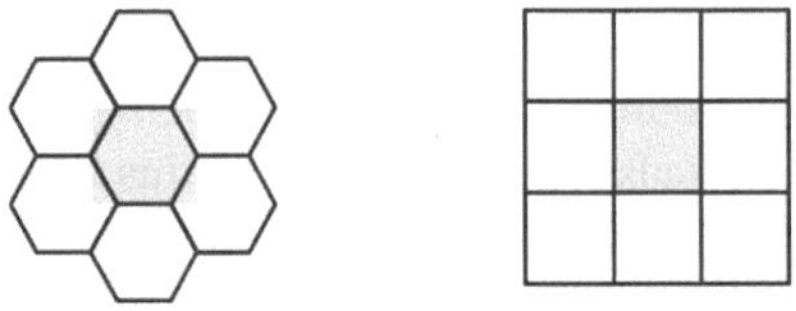

Fig. 4.31. The structuring element (a unit radius circle) on a hexagonal grid (left) and a square grid (right)

The general algorithm of a morphology transformation is as follows:

- The structuring element is moved around the whole image and for every point of the image, the image points are compared with the structuring element, assuming that the analyzed image point represents the central point of the structuring element;
- In every point of the image, it is checked whether the actual configuration of image pixels around this point is consistent with the structuring element pattern;
- If the pattern of pixels in the image and in the structuring element coincide, a specific operation is performed on the point analyzed (this usually consists in the "agreed" point being removed from the image, or conversely, added to it).

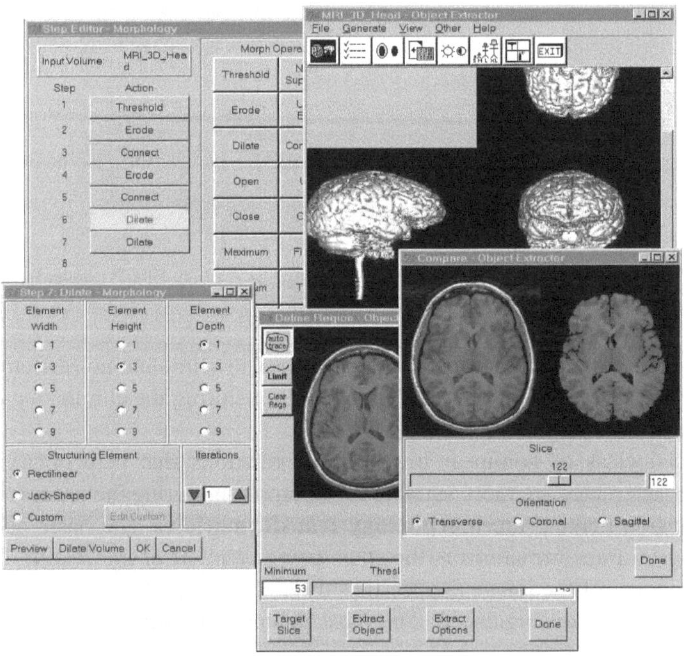

Fig. 4.32. An example of a tool for the morphology processing of medical images (source Internet)

Morphology transformations are widely used for medical images (see Fig. 4.32) due to their ability to very subtly handle the images being processed, which can be very important for the final result in the case of medical images.

We will now briefly discuss several basic morphology operations on medical images. The first one is **erosion.**

To define the operation of erosion, it is assumed that there is an irregular shape X and a circle B with the radius of r, which is the structuring element. The centre of circle B is taken as the central point of the structuring element. Then, the erosion of figure X with element B can be defined in two ways:

- The eroded figure is a set of all centers of circles with the radius of r which can completely fit inside area X;
- Circle B is rolled around the ***inside*** of the edge of the figure, and the subsequent positions of the centre of circle B plot the edge of the eroded figure (Fig. 4.33).

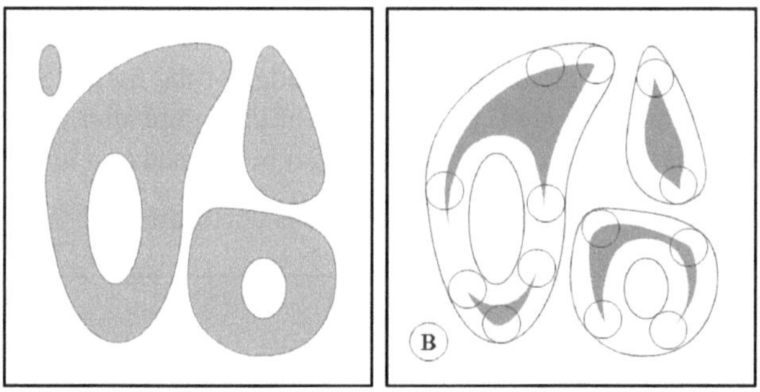

Fig. 4.33. An example of eroding (on the left: the image prior to eroding, on the right: the image after erosion and the structuring element used to erode it (a small circle marked with the B symbol))

Erosion can also be defined as the so-called minimum filter, i.e. an operator in which every point is assigned the ***minimum*** of the values of its neighbors.

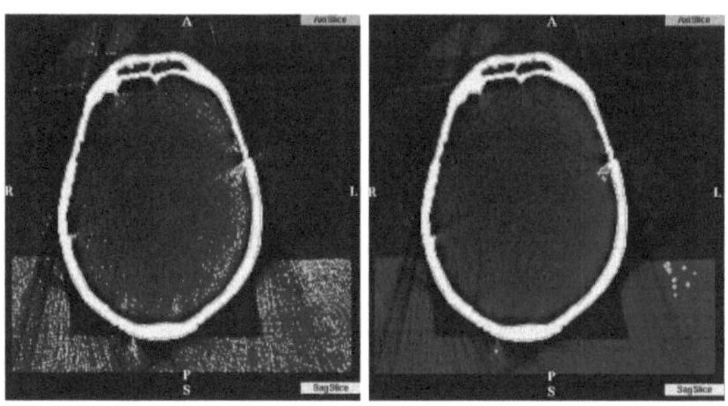

Fig. 4.34. Using erosion to remove interference from a medical image of skull bones

Erosion represents a very effective method of removing minor interference, which sometimes appears as the so-called apparatus artifacts in some medical images. This is illustrated by Fig. 4.34, which shows the original image on the left, and the image obtained by eroding it on the right. One feature of erosion is the **irrecoverable** removal of some small objects from the image (these are most frequently the above artifacts) which may be beneficial if we are convinced that those small objects constitute interference, but can be risky if the analyzed object itself contains small details which may be material from the point of view of its identification.

Dilatation (frequently called **dilation**) is exactly the opposite of erosion. To define the operation of dilatation, it is assumed there the image contains an irregular area (figure) X and a circle B with the radius of r, which represents the structuring element. Then, the dilatation of figure X with element B can be defined in three ways:

- Following the dilatation, the figure is a set of centers of all B circles which have at least one point overlapping with any point of the output figure,
- Circle B is rolled along the **outer side** of the edge of the figure. Subsequent locations of the centre of circle B plot the edge of the figure after dilatation;
- Just as in the case of the erosion, dilatation can be defined as a ***maximum filter.***

Fig. 4.35 shows an example of how dilatation is performed.

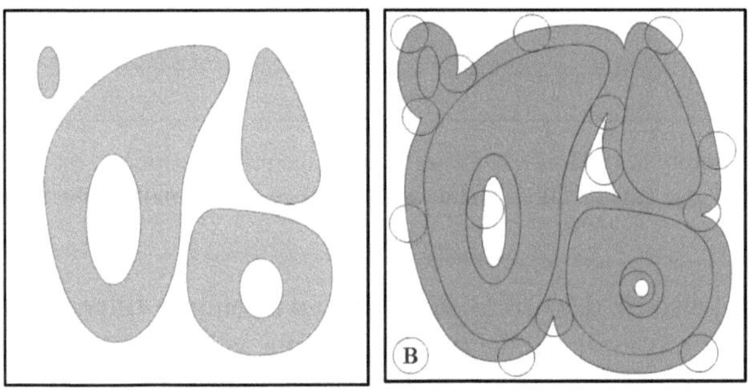

Fig. 4.35. An example of performing dilatation. Description as for Fig. 4.33

Transformations such as erosion and dilatation have a major shortcoming. They clearly change the surface area of the image transformed. This area is reduced by erosion and increased by dilatation. To eliminate this shortcoming, two transformations have been introduced which combine the above operations. These are referred to as **opening** and **closure,** and can be defined as follows:

opening = erosion + dilatation
closure = dilatation + erosion

Results of applying those combined operations are shown in Figures 4.36 and 4.37.

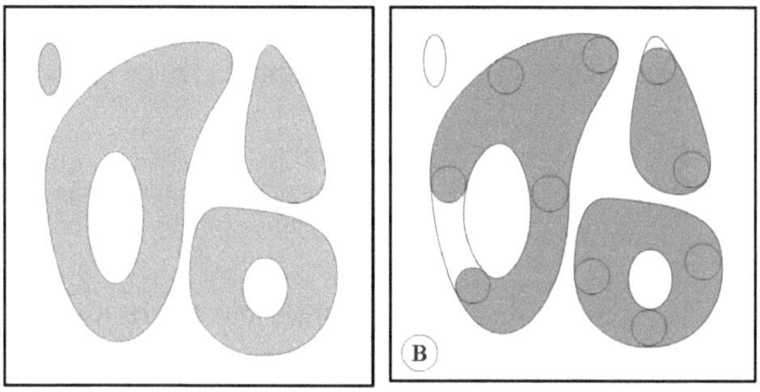

Fig. 4.36. An example of conducting the operation of opening. Description as in Fig. 4.33

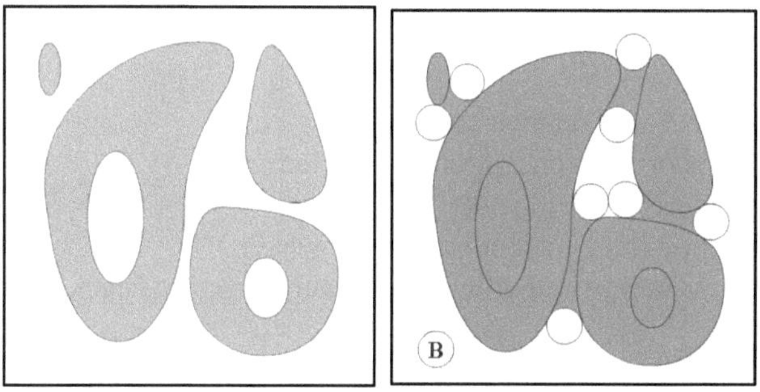

Fig. 4.37. An example of conducting the operation of closure. Description as in Fig. 4.33

Specialists have conflicting opinions of the suitability of the above operations for medical images. Some experts believe that operations of opening and closure enable modeling the image in a very subtle way, significantly improving its legibility, while others are of the opposite opinion. An argument supporting the second opinion is provided by Figure 4.38, which presents the effect of the morphology operation of opening conducted several times on a medical image. The operation was conducted to separate the image of the brain from eyeballs, but it resulted in breaking the connection between the areas and losing the precision.

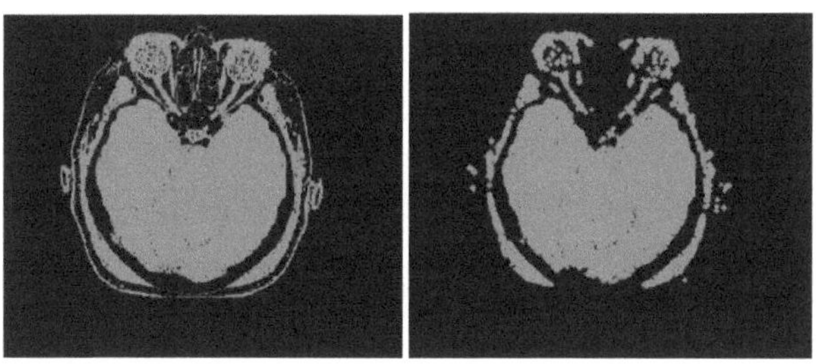

Fig. 4.38. The effect of several repetitions of the morphology operation of opening performed on the tomogram of the brain and eyeballs

Another morphology transformation – **skeletonizing** – is less controversial as to it suitability. Skeletonizing is an operation which allows axial points (skeletons) of figures to be distinguished in the analyzed image. Its more formal definition reads as follows:

The skeleton of a figure is the set of all points equidistant from at least two points belonging to the edge of the figure.

The skeleton of a figure is much smaller than that figure itself, but it gives a complete reflection of its basic topological characteristics. Figure 4.39 shows an example of skeletonization a pancreatic duct revealed in an ERCP examination, while Figure 4.40 explains the most popular skeletonization algorithm introduced by Pavlidis [45].

Examining figure skeletons supports analyses of medical images which include:

- Classifying cells based on their shapes;
- Determining the orientation of elongated objects;
- Separating "objects stuck together";
- Plotting the centre line of wider bands (e.g. vessels);
- Simulating processes of cell growth and grainy structure development.

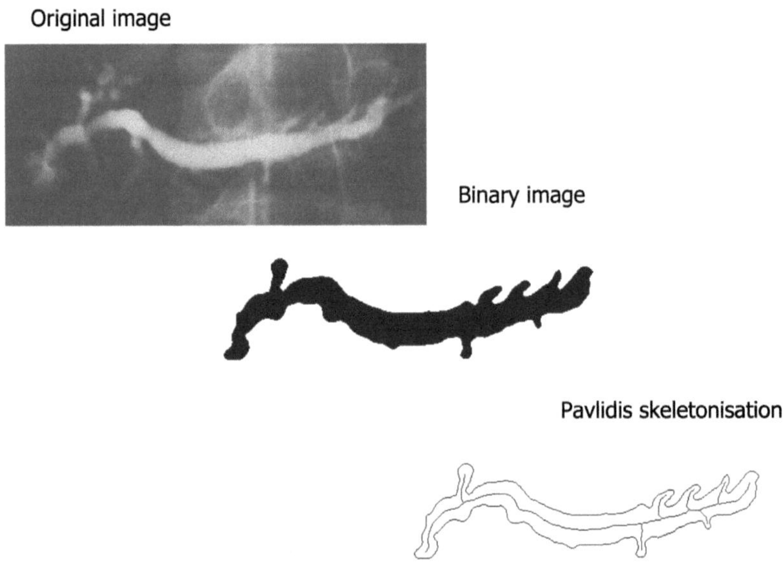

Fig. 4.39. An example of using skeletonization to analyze a medical image

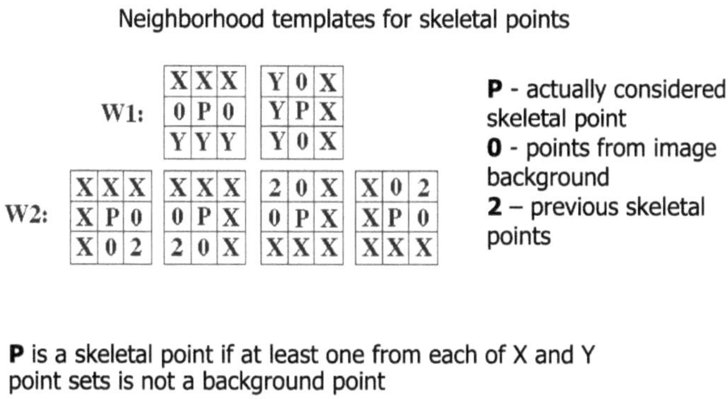

Fig. 4.40. The classical Pavlidis skeletonization algorithm

4.5. Binarization of medical images

4.5.1. General remarks

Segmentation usually represents the first step of the preliminary stage of medical image analysis. It allows material elements of the image of the organs examined to be distinguished while hiding the superfluous elements of the background. Its purpose is to significantly reduce the information content of the image and remove components which are immaterial from the point of view of semantic analysis. The segmentation process consists in converting the entire range of the grey scale (or colors) of a given image into an image that consists of only two colors, represented in a binary form as black and white. It is usually possible to use several binarizing methods, including the simplest methods of standard thresholding and advanced techniques aimed at segmenting complicated visualizations. Examples of more advanced methods will be described in subsequent chapters. Among the simplest binarization methods, it is worth noting the so-called binarization with a lower or upper threshold. These are defined as follows:

- Binarization with a lower threshold:

$$L' = \begin{cases} 0; L(m,n) \leq a \\ 1; L(m,n) > a \end{cases}$$

- Binarization with an upper threshold:

$$L' = \begin{cases} 0; L(m,n) \geq a \\ 1; L(m,n) < a \end{cases}$$

where:

L(m, n) – the brightness of the point in the source image; L(m, n) ={0,1,2, ...,255}

L'(m, n) – the value of that point in the output image, which can be either 0 or 255;

a – the binarization threshold.

When using this method, it is necessary to select the binarization threshold. One of the simplest ways of selecting that threshold is to analyze the histogram [47], which shows the distribution of the number of image points of a specific grey level.

Figure 4.41 shows an example of an ERCP image of the pancreatic duct and its histogram, as well as the results of running a simple thresholding of the grey level specified in the histogram.

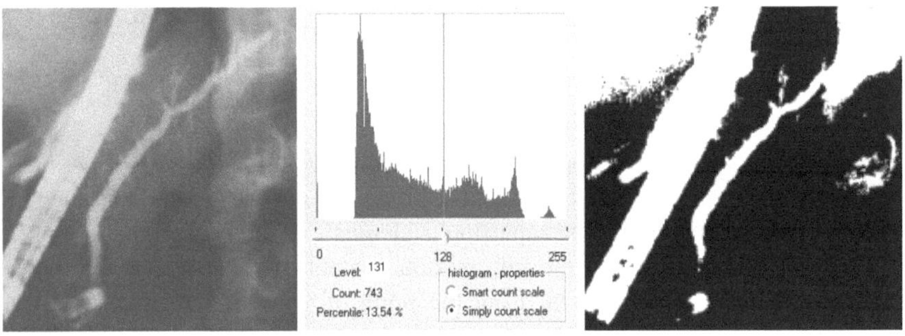

Fig. 4.41. A) The original ERCP image in grey levels. B) Image histogram with a binarization threshold set at 131. C) Image after binarizing

If images contain objects whose grey levels are much different from image background elements, such simple methods as binarization with a single threshold may yield satisfactory results. Unfortunately, in most cases, they leave too many unimportant elements, so other, more advanced and orientated methods are frequently needed. Such somewhat more advanced methods of image binarization allow images to be segmented.

Image segmentation will be analyzed in more detail in the next chapter (chapter 5) of this book, while here we will only define it as dividing an image into regions of specific characteristics. The result of a simple binarization or a more advanced segmentation of medical images is to segregate objects specific for the patient and dependent on the type of examination (the heart, the liver, kidneys, lungs, the brain etc.). In general, the right segmentation method should be selected depending on the type of images processed, the expected results and their subsequent analysis. Not every segmentation method will turn out to be suitable for a given image type but the effects of various segmentation algorithms can frequently be combined, so that masking and logical operations on binary images can be used. Such combinations frequently yield satisfactory results.

It has already been mentioned that segmentation will be discussed in greater detail in a separate chapter devoted to that subject. However, as segmentation is connected with the binarization that we are discussing here, we should note that the following binarization techniques can be distinguished:

4.5.2. Binarization by simple thresholding

Binarization by thresholding has been described above as consisting in setting a threshold value, i.e. a specific grey level which marks the border between the image background and objects. As a result of this process, all points of the image which are less bright than the threshold value will be assigned the value of zero, for example, while points whose brightness is at least equal to the threshold value will receive the maximum value. This kind of binarizing can be executed with two or more threshold values.

If there are two thresholds, points with a brightness between the thresholds are assigned the logical value of one and are classified as the object, while the remaining points are assigned the logical value of zero and classified as the background. The thresholds can be selected by way of an experiment, e.g. by analyzing the source histogram, or automatically by a computer application based on certain heuristics. A special type of segmentation by thresholding is the segmentation of color images by creating chromatic masks, in which three monochromatic images corresponding to primary colors are extracted from the color image, and then thresholds are set for each channel. The points whose brightness in every channel is between the thresholds are assigned the logical value of one, and the remaining points – of zero.

4.5.3. Binarization by detecting edges

Binarization by detecting edges is a method consisting in determining the gradients of the image, and one possible way of doing so is by using gradient (high pass) filters which enhance all object edges, or directional edges. The image obtained in this fashion is not a purely binary image, but the edges feature a certain brightness distribution. To unanimously determine object edges, it is necessary to define the criterion of the image point belonging to the object edge. Such criteria include analyzing different brightness gradients in a defined neighborhood of every point. If this difference is greater than a certain threshold value, then the point is considered to belong to the border of the object. For such methods, we can define parameters such as the size of the area of the neighborhood considered and the threshold of gradients used for locally describing image contrasts. Every area with a contrast greater than the threshold is treated as the object and assigned the logical value of one. Such operations aimed at detecting edges are frequently referred to as a dynamic or adaptive segmentation. It should be noted that this segmentation process only determines the borders of structures, while the area inside these borders is empty and has the logical value of zero. Also watershed detection and many other gradient algorithms, like Roberts, Canny, Sobel, Prewitt etc. [28, 48] are classified as edge detection methods.

4.5.4. Binarization by region growing

Binarization, or more generally segmenting by growing consists in grouping points or fragments of an image into larger regions. The course of this process consists in looking around initial pixels for other pixels which fulfill a predefined similarity condition. That condition may specify the brightness, color and texture. If a given point fulfills the predefined condition, it is added to the region while the similarity criterion is applied to neighboring points: if they also fulfill the criterion, they are added to the region. If no point adjacent to the region meets the condition, region growth ends. Depending on the number of regions into which the image is to be split, the appropriate number of initial points is selected [47, 48].

4.5.5. Binarization with the use of neuron networks

These techniques consist in assigning points or fragments of an image to one of the predefined pattern classes (for binarization, these are two classes, labeled as 0 and 1, but more generally there may be more classes). Classification is performed by an appropriately trained neuron network which can take an image fragment and a set of features defined for a specific fragment as the input data. On the output, that network generates the number of the class to which a given image fragment or point has been assigned. MLP feed forward networks, Kohonen self-organizing networks and Hopfield recurrent networks are most commonly used [48].

4.6. Hough transform in medical applications

In an analysis of medical images we should also mention the Hough transform [48], proposed by Paul Hough in 1962. The transform is a special case of the Radon transform known since 1917, which is equivalent to the Hough transform for binary images. The main purpose of the transform is to extract regular sets of points forming lines, circles, arcs etc. from the image. To analyze the notion behind the Hough transform for the simplest example of identifying a straight line in an image, a set of collinear points should be determined in the image using the following formula:

$$\lambda_0 = \{(x, y) \in R^2 : y - ax - b = 0\}$$

where a and b are parameters characterizing the straight line. The solution of this equation is a set of points on a plane, the characteristic feature of that set being that for one point we can obtain a set of collinear points in the parameter space. This facilitates determining all straight lines bisecting the point and then selecting those straight lines which might cause the pixel searched for to become active. Determining the appropriate straight lines is closely linked with the notion of reverse protection, which consists in analyzing every active pixel of the image to identify those straight lines.

Figure 4.42 shows the graphic representation of a linear Hough transform. That transform maps the Cartesian plane to a two-dimensional plane of parameters (ρ,Θ) describing straight lines (a Hough plane). The straight line from the Cartesian plane is mapped to a single point in the Hough plane, the coordinates of that point unambiguously identifying that straight line. A point from the Cartesian plane is represented in the Hough plane by a sinusoidal curve that identifies a set of straight lines bisecting the same point: see the formula below.

$$x^*cos\,\theta_0 + y^*sin\,\theta_0 = \rho_0 \;\rightarrow\; (\rho_0,\ \theta_0)$$

$$(x_0,\ y_0) \rightarrow x_0^*cos\,\theta + y_0^*sin\,\theta = \rho,\ 0 \leq \theta < 2\pi \qquad (4.1)$$

Relationship (4.1) indicates that the point where two curves representing the transforms of two different Cartesian space points intersect in the Hough space identifies the straight line which bisects both of these points in the Cartesian space (Fig. 4.42).

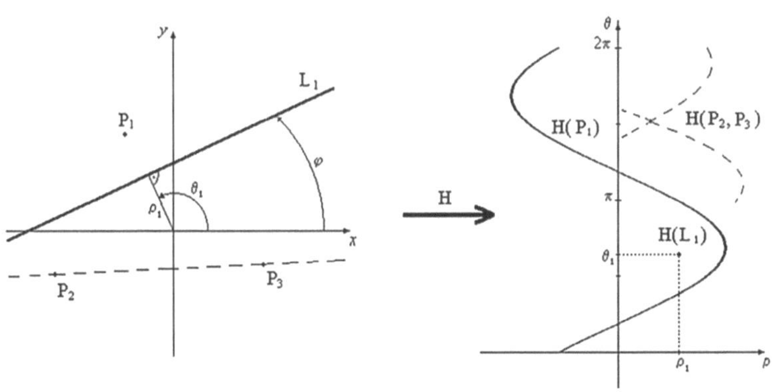

Fig. 4.42. A graphic representation of the Hough transform. An example of mapping the straight line L1 and points P1, P2 and P3 from a Cartesian plane to a Hough plane. A) Cartesian space, B) Hough transform space

Using this transform to process digital images consists in finding a point in the transformed image, in which point a large number of curves representing points of the Cartesian space intersect. This point may mean that the original image contains a straight section belonging to the straight line mapped to a point in the Hough space. This point is where sinusoids intersect in the transformed image – Fig. 4.42.B. The real appearance of the Hough space for an image in which three clear lines can be detected (among other things) is shown in Fig. 4.43.

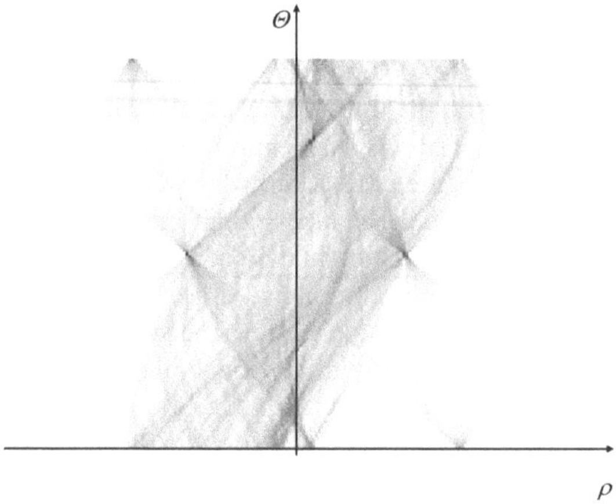

Fig. 4.43. The real appearance of the Hough space

Several types of Hough transforms are distinguished, the main ones including:

1. a fast Hough transform;
2. a probabilistic Hough transform;
3. a randomized Hough transform;
4. a hierarchical Hough transform;
5. a fuzzy Hough transform; and
6. a variable resolution transform.

Practical problems most frequently solved using the Hough method include not just identifying straight lines, but also curves, arcs, polygons, circles or ellipses, but the ability to apply this method to 3D images is also being considered.

To calculate the Hough transform using a computer we need the correct representation of the parameter space. Every dimension of it is narrowed and quantized at the selected precision level. This applies to the values of variables (ρ, Θ). As a result, we get an array called the accumulator in which every element is identified by its respective (quantized) values of parameters.

The Hough transform has many advantages. As every point of the image is treated independently, it can be executed using parallel calculations and multiprocessor systems, which means that it is suitable for real time systems. This method is relatively independent of image interference (due to quantizing the values of angles and distances of straight lines) so it can recognize even somewhat distorted objects. Frequently, even if only 5% – 15% of pixels from the image are available, it can be used to detect an object in the image, as well as circles, spheres and ellipses.

The Hough transform also has drawbacks, of which the main one is the large memory demand of the accumulator and the significant computational complexity.

5. Algorithms and methods for the goal-oriented processing of medical images

This chapter contains a brief description of non-standard operations of medical image processing and analysis used for specialized analyses aimed at developing semantic descriptions of recognized patterns.

5.1. Segmentation of medical images

One of the key stages in medical image analysis is the binarization or the segmentation of the images under consideration. Among the numerous well-known methods of simple binarizing described in Section 4.5, we can also distinguish dedicated contour separation algorithms developed particularly for specific types of medical images. Such proposals frequently include methods based on various sorts of heuristics. This section will present two selected examples of heuristic segmentation algorithms dedicated to separating contours in X-ray and USG images. The first one is a method which allows one to separate the contours of gallbladders in USG images [6], the second is for determining the edges of pancreatic ducts in ERCP (*Endoscopic Retrograde Cholangiopancreatography*) images [27].

The purpose for which medical images are segmented is always to distinguish from the whole image those elements (usually the outlines of the organs under consideration – Figure 5.1) which are then to be further analyzed. An object distinguished as a result of segmenting can then be subjected to detailed analyses without any clutter due to the need to take other objects into account. Segmentation is also useful if the medical image, after its processing, will be visually assessed by physicians, and becomes indispensable if the next processing stage is automatic image interpretation, and particularly automatic image understanding.

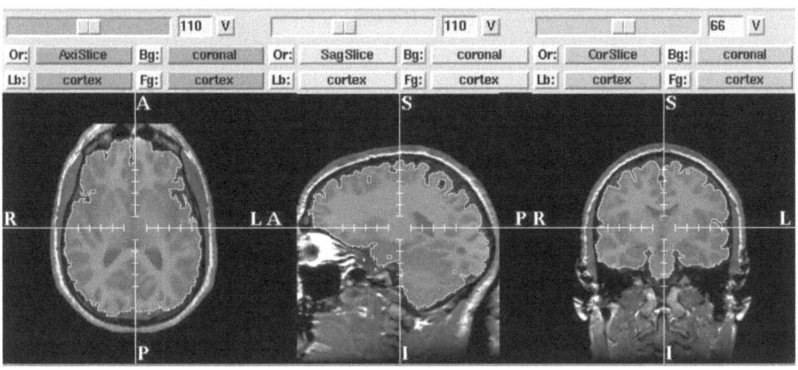

Fig. 5.1. An example of a segmentation distinguishing the object of interest (here: the patient's brain) from the whole image (source Internet)

M.R. Ogiela and R. Tadeusiewicz: *Algorithms and methods for the goal-oriented processing of medical images,* Studies in Computational Intelligence (SCI) **84**, 99–115 (2007)
www.springerlink.com

Segmentation should distinguish the object to be analyzed using the simplest means possible, so if it is possible to formulate a simple definition of the difference between the shape (for example) of objects examined and those that are not, this simplest possible criterion should be used. Figure 5.2 shows the microscopic image of a semen sample. The goal of its segmentation is to distinguish the contours of sperm in this image, to later determine (further along in the analysis) how many of them are of the proper form, and how many exhibit defects.

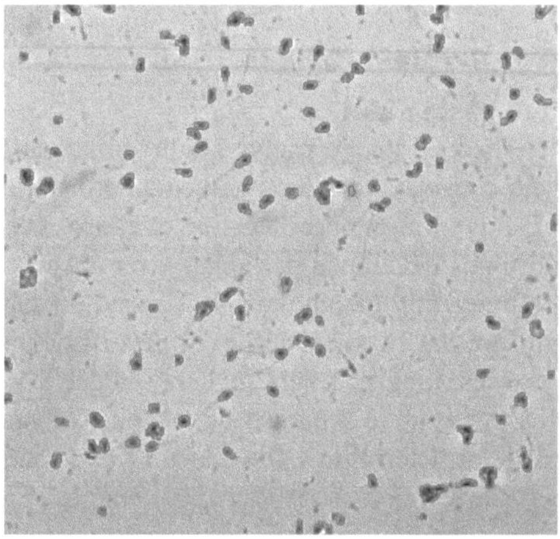

Fig. 5.2. An image of a semen sample showing the results of its segmentation aimed at distinguishing the contours of sperm for their further analysis

For this simple segmentation type, aimed at distinguishing relatively uncomplicated objects in the image, a simple algorithm consisting of just a few uncomplicated rules can be used (Figure 5.3).

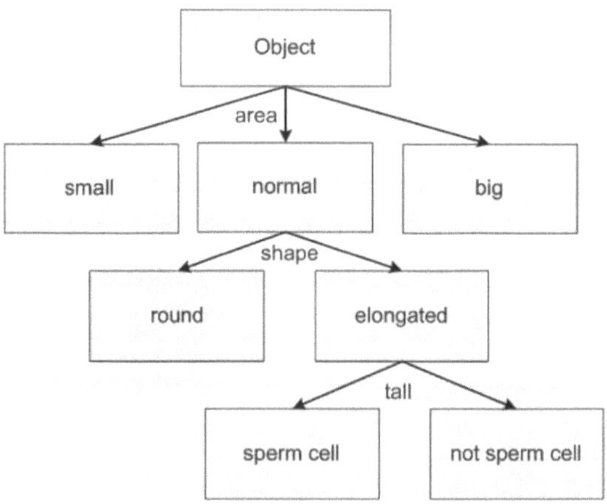

Fig. 5.3. An example of a simple set of rules used for the segmentation shown in Fig. 5.2

In the case of very many segmentation jobs applied to medical image, the object to be segmented is quite significantly different from other objects featured in the image, for example due to its brightness level (Fig. 5.4).

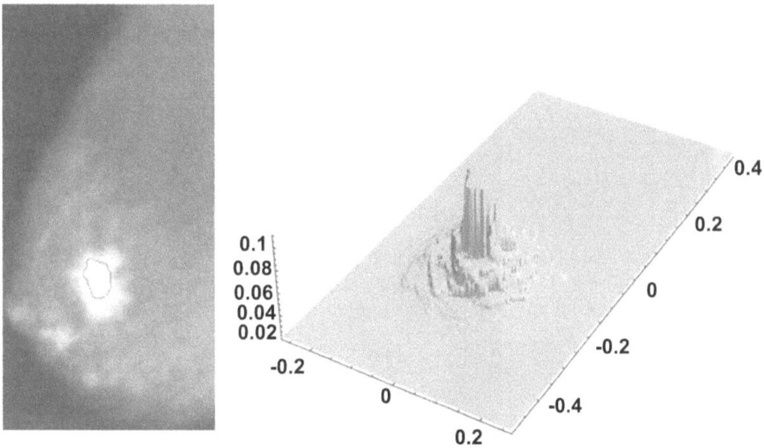

Fig. 5.4. This segmentation job is easy as the object to be distinguished (a tumor in the nipple area) differs from its surroundings in its brightness (visible in the chart on the right) (source Internet)

If objects to be distinguished differ from their surroundings in their brightness or color, the segmentation job really boils down to just selecting the right image thresholding, although in this case the selection of the threshold may determine how many of what details will be detected in the image segmented (Figure 5.5).

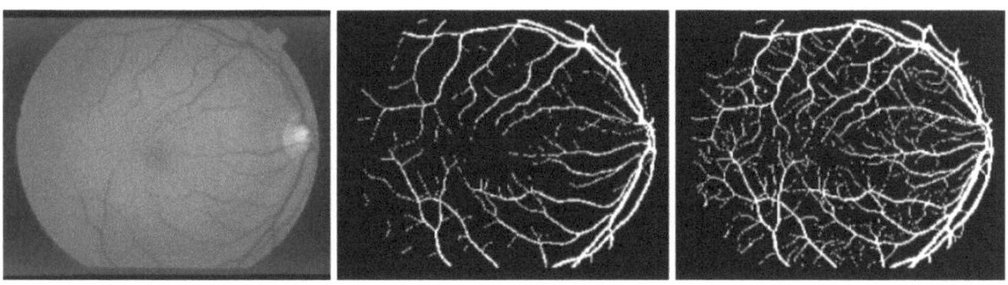

Fig. 5.5. Depending on the segmentation threshold selected, the segmentation can be run so as to distinguish more or less details of the object being distinguished

As it is difficult for physicians to set the segmentation criteria, sometimes the analyzed images are segmented semi-automatically (using a dialogue with the user). The sequence of steps in such a dialogue system is presented in Figure 5.6. First, the doctor indicates a characteristic (in his opinion) fragment of the image under consideration, which contains the structure of interest (see Fig. 5.6 on the left). The computer uses this as the basis for determining segmentation criteria and shows an image of the object distinguished from the image as a result of this segmentation (see Fig. 5.6, in the middle). When the doctor approves that it was really that object he/she had in mind and that its borders have been defined properly, the computer defines the search criteria and analyses the entire image to distinguish and pinpoint other objects which meet the same criteria, and so are probably of interest to the physician (see Fig. 5.6, right side).

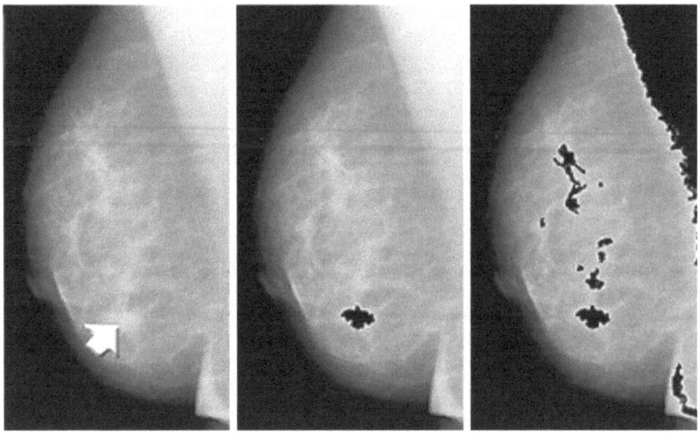

Fig. 5.6. A dialogue procedure for the medical image segmentation process. Explained in the text

In more complicated jobs, the problem of distinguishing the object under analysis can be somewhat more complicated. It often happens that image fragments with the same optical density (grey level) must be segmented separately (Fig. 5.7).

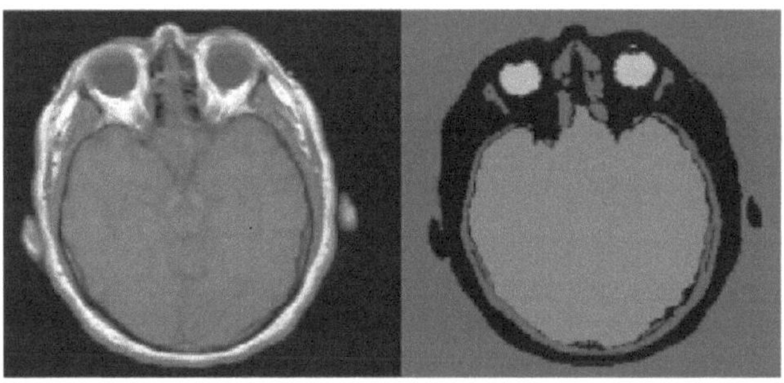

Fig. 5.7. During a segmentation aimed at distinguishing one anatomical structure (here: the brain), structures with the same characteristics (eyes) can pose a problem

5.2. Segmentation based on the image texture

Apart from the simple segmentation methods described above, which mainly differentiate grey levels and are dedicated to specific types of medical images, another frequent solution uses the **texture** as the factor distinguishing the object to be analyzed from the elements (arbitrarily!) classified as the insignificant background. This is justified, because the methods and ways of acquiring medical images have been chosen by all the inventors and designers mentioned in Chapter 2 so that differences in biological properties of the tissues imaged could be observed as differences between the features of acquired images, including differences in their texture.

Unlike simple features such as image brightness or its grey level, texture can be relatively easy to visually notice in the image, but is difficult to describe in terms of parameters that can be determined by a computer during digital image processing. Further on in our considerations, we will use algorithms classified to one of four classes of texture segmentation methods. The classes are as follows [6]:

1. Statistical approaches which analyze object texture in quantitative terms. Some correlations of color (or grey level) distribution are also analyzed in two and multi-dimensional images (e.g. the scattering of characteristic points or their concentrations). Statistical approaches do not aim at describing the structure of the image analyzed, but at calculating the parameters of statistical position measures such as the histogram, the mean, the variance, the asymmetry (slope) or the kurtosis (the measure of how flat the distribution of a characteristic is).
2. Structural methods, which examine the structure of constituent elements of images, relatively small compared to the whole image. These elements are called microtextures (patterns), and their distribution in the plane is referred to as the macrotexture. In this case, to make a structural description of the texture, two factors are necessary: the definition of the microtexture and the rules of its distribution in the image. The description of the microtexture can take any shape, from a pattern in the form of a sequence of symbols defining textures, to a graph description of the microtexture. When such patterns are compared to the information contained in the derivative rules of image grammars, patterns can be detected which correspond to strictly defined shapes.
3. Transform methods, based on mapping the analyzed image fragment, treated as a Cartesian plane, to another space. This transform is to amplify the features significant for texture classification. For example, the Fourier transform supports the frequency analysis of the image, while the Hough transform is widely used to analyze images containing sections of straight lines (e.g. the analysis of bone trabeculation images).
4. Model based methods use fractal or stochastic models to interpret the image. The most widely used are image generative models (e.g. those forming the basis of algorithms of fractal image compression) or stochastic models, such as Markov random fields (MRF).

These methods, when used separately for specific images, usually do not yield satisfactory results. However, their combinations sometimes allow the area of a biological structure of interest to us to be distinguished. As these methods are not always able to yield unanimous information on the edges of the analyzed structures, the are used in combinations. However, even after their combination, their success always depends on the type of medical image being examined. This is why dedicated procedures, developed especially to enable an effective analysis of specific types of images, are frequently used to unanimously identify the object we need in the examined image. Further down in the chapter we will present two examples of such algorithms. The first one helps in segmenting USG gallbladder images, and the second is dedicated to segmenting ERCP X-rays of the pancreas.

5.3. Separating gallbladders from USG images

One of the most difficult types of medical images subjected to computer processing, including the stages of automatic segmentation, are USG images of soft tissues and internal organs. The difficulties in segmenting such images are mainly due to the neighboring structures (imaged using the USG) having similar acoustic resistance and echogenic properties, and therefore taking similar grey levels in the images acquired. This makes this type of images difficult to segment and forces us to find dedicated methods for their analysis.

This chapter presents a heuristic algorithm proposed by S. Bodzioch [6, 7] which enables successfully separating the contours of a gallbladder shown in USG images. This algorithm is based on combining the results of two independent segmentations of such images, made using a rank filter and a method for analyzing secants determined for the gallbladder under examination.

The first stage – rank filtering – enables potential edges, which are fragments of gallbladder walls, to be detected. The structures detected in the image (potential gallbladder walls) are smoothed out and joined into a continuous whole by the repeated execution of a transform using a rank filter. This yields an image containing continuous, smooth lines, which may form parts of the organ being separated (Fig. 5.8). The second stage of this processing, running in parallel, is to separate the contour by using the algorithm of analyzing histogram secants for the organ examined. In the end, once the results of both of these independent procedures have been obtained, it becomes possible to merge the results into one final image which shows the separated contours of the gallbladder.

The general diagram of how this procedure works is shown in Figure 5.8. We will now take a somewhat closer look at the procedure of some component operations which make up the conceptual diagram of this algorithm.

In this algorithm, the rank filtering stage consists of 3 steps. These are:

1. The binarization;
2. Using the rank filter to filter the binary image;
3. Determining the contour of borders between areas of different colors.

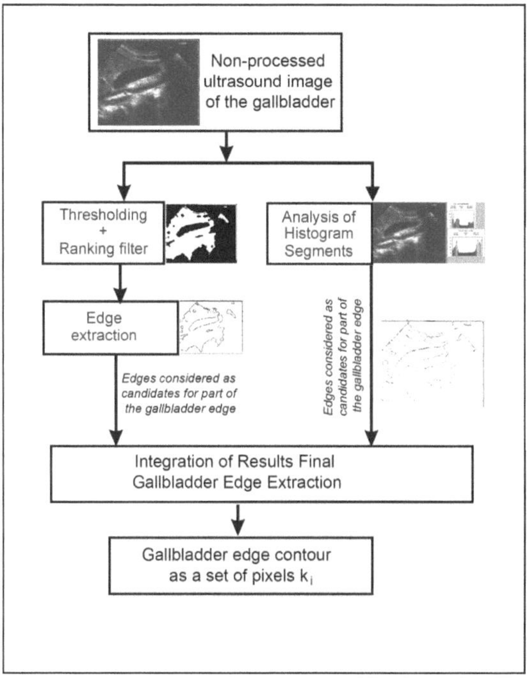

Fig. 5.8. An algorithm for extracting GB walls from ultrasound images

At the binarizing stage, the segmentation threshold selection is calculated separately for each analyzed image (dynamic selection). This is done as follows: first the mean of colors (grey levels) of the whole image is calculated, and then the mean minus 10 (this is an empirically selected value [7]) is taken as the binarizing threshold.

In the next algorithm step, the rank filter is used. In this filtering, it is assumed that every pixel of the image will be assigned the black color if within the surroundings of this pixel having the radius of 2 there are 13 or more black pixels. (13 is another experimentally established value [6].) If the above method is adopted, the filter can process the image multiple times, until it reaches a balance at which the image stops changing after another iteration. This transform is repeated 10 times (this value has also been selected experimentally) and leads to a significant improvement in the quality of this image. During studies conducted using the proposed algorithm, we observed the filling of "bay-type" fragments of the image, the removal of small groups of black pixels called "islands", and a general smoothing of lines which represent presumed contours of gallbladder walls. Due to these characteristics of the rank filter, the edges of areas determined by image binarization are smoothed and filtered from single isolated pixels.

The last step of this branch of the algorithm is edge detection. In the processed image, at the border of two areas of different color, only a black line (2 pixels wide) of the contour is left, while the remaining areas are left white. This is a transform that checks whether within the surroundings of the point having the radius of one there are points of the opposite color, and if there are, the point is changed to black. If there are none, the color of the point is changed to white.

The above steps yield images which can be compared to those obtained from the other algorithm branch. These images are recorded in the system as ones subjected to preliminary segmentation by rank filtering. However, the proper final results of the segmentation are only generated by merging these images with images created by the procedure of edge detection using secants, which is described below.

The secant method is based on the histogram analysis. In an analysis of histograms of pixel grey levels, generated for pixels which belong to the secants running across the gallbladder image in different directions (see Figure 5.9), the gallbladder walls are shown as the local extremes of those histograms. Details of analyses of such extremes are given in source publication [6]. The only important element of this analysis is that it allows us to independently detect points which may form the contour of the structure being analyzed.

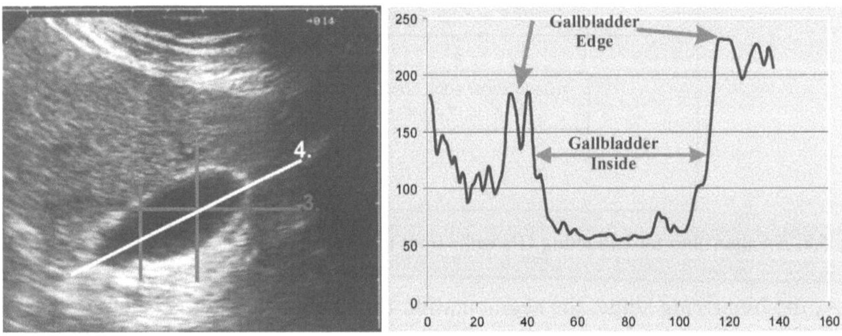

Fig. 5.9. A sample histogram analysis of digital image sections, A) The analyzed image with analyzed sections marked in red, B) A histogram graph of Segment 1 [6]

As the transforms described above yield two separate images, the next stage is to merge them into a single image containing only those edges which really form parts of the organ walls, while the remaining ones should be removed. The stage of integrating partial results of the above edge detection procedures is illustrated in Figure 5.10. The details of this procedure are described in source publication [7].

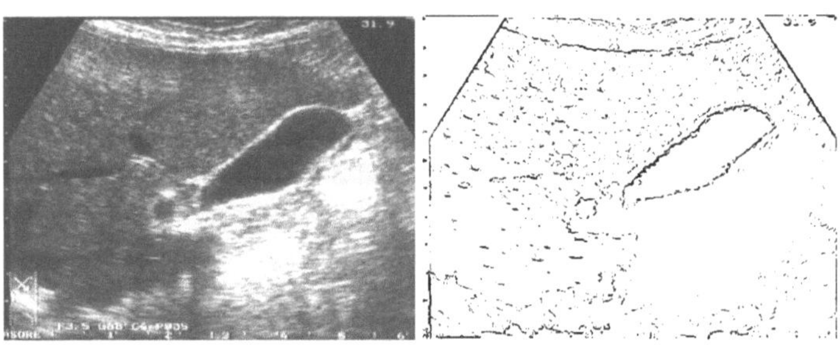

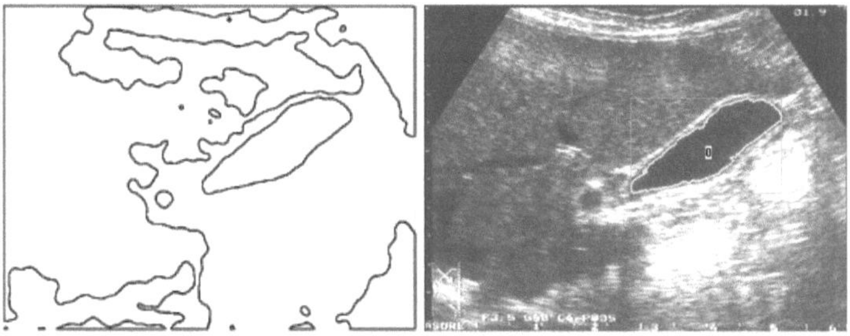

C) D)

Fig. 5.10. An example of intermediate images generated by integrating outcome images of gallbladder edge extraction algorithms for a single case, A) An ultrasound image of a healthy gallbladder, B) An ultrasound image of a gallbladder filtered using the method of analyzing horizontal and vertical secants, C) An ultrasound image of a gallbladder filtered using the method based on a rank filter, D) An ultrasound image of a healthy gallbladder with the detected organ contour marked

The procedure described above has turned out to be extremely successful, as its effectiveness of detecting gallbladder walls exceeds 90% [6] which should be considered a very good result, particularly in the view of the poor legibility of the input image.

5.4. Segmenting ERCP images

Another example of an adaptive segmentation procedure is the procedure for extracting the outline of the shape of contrast-filled pancreatic ducts (the main duct and sometimes the additional one), shown during ERCP examinations, from the whole X-ray image.

We can quote one successful method of segmenting such images, proposed by Mikrut in publication [27]. Authors' research has proven the utility of that algorithm, which has been selected as the optimum binarizing method not just for ERCP images, but also for segmenting coronarography images, urograms, and tomograms of the spinal cord [55].

The formal description of this algorithm is presented in publication [27], so here we will only qualitatively characterize the idea behind it. It works in the following way:

During the binarization of the image under analysis, this method determines the edge points of the examined structure that are looked for (e.g. of the vessel to be distinguished) by analyzing the derivatives of eight scalar functions. These functions have been defined as densitometry profiles of eight directional straight lines shown in Fig. 5.11.

Directional straight lines form a symmetrical star of canonical directions and all begin in the so-called *central analysis points* (automatically selected in subsequent binarization stages). When selecting subsequent central analysis points, we take into account all points which belong to their direct or somewhat more distant neighborhood. The first central analysis point must be indicated manually (so that the algorithm will know which of the many anatomical structures it is to distinguish). If the process of filling the analyzed vessel with the contrast medium was not properly conducted or if the advanced disease process has led to a very significant stenosis of the vessel's opening in some of its sections, the outline of the vessel in the X-ray may be discontinuous. If so, it is necessary to manually indicate, in the binarizing program, at least one initial central analysis point in every clearly visible segment of the anatomical structure under consideration.

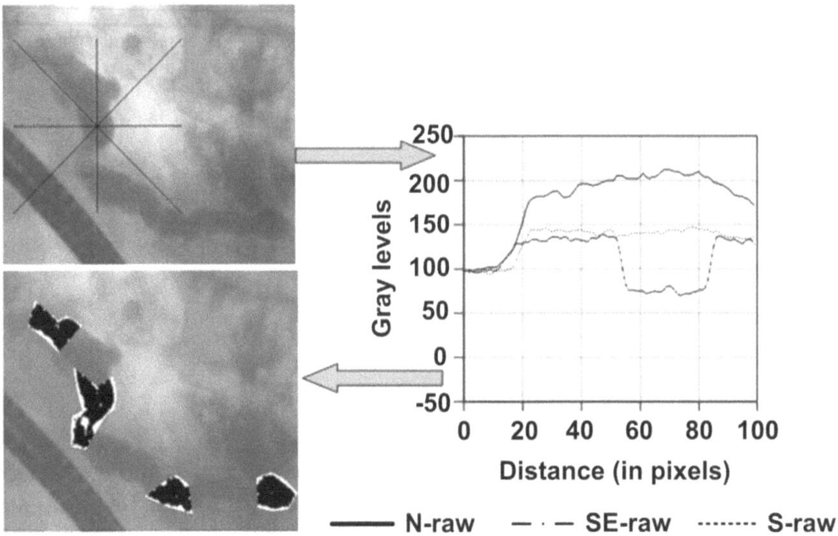

Fig. 5.11. A dedicated algorithm for thresholding ERCP images [27]

The densitometry functions introduced identify changes in grey levels of subsequent image points along defined directional straight lines, depending on their distance from the central analysis point currently analyzed. The point in which a high negative value of the derivative of the current densitometric function is observed is selected as an edge point, but this decision is additionally verified by the context (using adjacent points, which should also include previously detected edge points). This way, image segmentation as well as the distinguishing (and binarizing) of the image of the inside of the vessel considered is performed in a distributed way (at the same time for many sections of the shown vessel): first in the areas where the natural contrast between the vessel and the surrounding tissue is particularly good, and only then in areas where that contrast is worse, but where contextual information from the known, previously extracted fragments of the contour can already be used. Details of this binarizing method (which has turned out to be very effective) are too complicated for their complete presentation here, but, as already mentioned, can be read in paper [27].

It is worth adding that this complex binarization procedure should be used only for particularly difficult images (like the image of a pancreatic duct poorly filled with the contrast medium and overlapping with the image of the spine). In the case of other, easier medical images, the right approach to segmenting and detecting the edges of the analyzed vessels is to use subtractive merging of original images with those subjected to high-pass filtering. The result of this operation should then be subjected to gradient analysis methods, which have been designed specifically to detect edges.

5.5. Thinning and skeletonizing objects in images

In the case of computer analyses of medical structures featuring complicated shapes or major morphological changes, it may be beneficial to **thin** or **skeletonize** the examined structures to identify changes in their shapes that will be useful for the further analysis. Such operations are necessary, for example, when analyzing tubular structures (vessels, the spinal cord, ureters) using the **straightening transform** described in the following section.

Both of these operations use the morphological structural elements defined for contextual image processing.

Thinning with the use of a structural element consists in overlaying that element over each point of the image in such a way that its central point coincides with the point being analyzed, and then executing either of the possible operations:

- Leaving the point unchanged if the structural element does not coincide with its neighborhood;
- Changing the value of the point, for example to 0, if the structural element fully fits the neighborhood of the analyzed point.

The thinning process can be run iteratively until subsequent steps no longer introduce significant changes to the image.

Skeletonizing represents a special case of the thinning process. Skeletonizing should yield the centre (skeleton) line of the thinned object, which line is equidistant from the external edges and one unit thick.

The skeletonizing algorithm should meet the following requirements:

- The skeleton should conserve the continuity and the shape of the original object;
- The skeleton should be located centrally and be equidistant from external edges of the object;
- The algorithm should not cause excessive erosion of the object, so that end points of the skeleton are detected as fast as possible, and so that the line which characterizes the object should not be excessively shortened compared to the actual length of the anatomical structure which that skeleton should represent;

– The skeleton should be independent of small perturbations of external edges of the processed object, while interferences and other external objects should have no impact on the shape of the skeleton.

The Pavlidis skeletonizing algorithm [45] can be used to skeletonize structures visible in medical images, as numerous research projects using real medical images have proven it to be the best (in terms of the stability of operation and the quality of the skeleton obtained) of the many known thinning algorithms [55].

This algorithm works as follows: any point P belonging to the object being thinned is removed from the image if the following criteria are met:

- P is an edge point (so at least one of its direct neighbors is a background point);
- P is not the end point;
- The neighborhood of point P does not correspond to any of the W1, W2 neighborhood patterns which define skeleton points of the object. The W1 and W2 patterns are defined as shown in Figure 5.12.

W1:

X	X	X
0	P	0
Y	Y	Y

Y	0	Y
Y	P	Y
Y	0	X

W2:

X	X	X
X	P	0
X	0	2

X	X	X
0	P	X
2	0	X

2	0	X
0	P	X
X	X	X

Fig. 5.12. Neighborhood patterns for skeleton points of the image in the Pavlidis method

In Figure 5.12 "P" denotes the point currently under consideration, **0** means points of the image background, and **2** represents skeleton points. Point P is a skeleton point if at least one of every group of X and Y points is different from the background, i.e. it belongs to the object or is already a skeleton point marked as 2.

The main advantage of this algorithm is that it generates continuous, very regular and smooth skeletons that are 1 unit wide and centrally located. Unlike in other frequently used algorithms, the lines it generates are also only negligibly shortened at the ends of the analyzed structure. A crucial advantage from the point of view of the effectiveness of further analysis is that the Pavlidis algorithm leaves the smallest number of apparent side branches in the skeleton, which are generated (as artifacts) by every skeletonizing process as a result of processing the unavoidable, small irregularities in the contours of the skeletonized anatomical structures.

An example result of skeletonizing a binary image showing a pancreatic duct exhibiting chronic inflammation symptoms is presented in Figure 5.13.

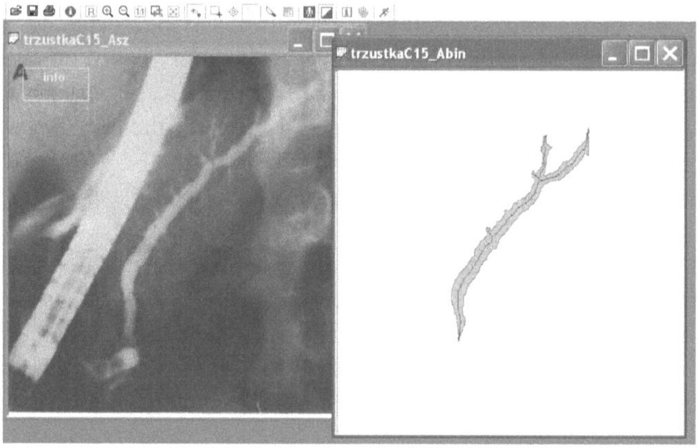

Fig. 5.13. An example of skeletonizing an image showing the pancreatic duct. The large structure visible on the left side of the image is not an anatomical structure, but a medical instrument (a duodenoscope) used to introduce the contrast medium

5.6. An example of a special type of medical image processing: the straightening transform

One of the most interesting proposals for non-standard transformations of objects in images is the **straightening transform** procedure proposed by the authors in publication [55] and then used in many subsequent studies. The use of this transform yields a new graphic representation of the medical structure being examined, much more suitable for analyzing its meaning. This is particularly useful to analyze structures of a tubular nature, as it allows changes in their morphology to be detected, making the analysis process independent of the spatial orientation of the examined organ in the image and its natural (individually variable) curvature. The characteristic feature of this procedure is that we use a sequence of geometrical conversions to transform the organ contour from a 2D image freely laid out in a plane to a 2D graph which, even though it maps the complex shape of the outline of the object under examination, is based on a central axis with the forced shape of a straight line. The width profiles of the examined structure obtained in this way present the contours of straightened organs together with the various internal changes that may occur in them, such as side branches, bulges, strictures and widenings, bifurcations of the structure or its amputations. The greatest advantage of this method is that it retains all the morphological changes which occur in the original organ, both those within the physiological norm and the pathological ones, of crucial importance during the formulation of the final diagnosis.

Graphs of structures thus obtained can then be subjected to a deeper analysis, recognition and classification, also using the syntactic methods of image recognition described in this book. The straightening transform has been applied to identify diseases, including the identification of pancreas disorders based on ERCP X-ray examinations, to analyze the condition of coronary vessels shown during coronarography examinations, to assess upper sections of the urinary tract as well as to interpret MRI images of the spinal cord.

In their most recent works, the authors have shown that this algorithm can also be used for the 3D analysis and modeling of spatially complex anatomical structures, including the organs of the abdominal cavity, or for reconstructing the bronchial/respiratory tree when identifying lung cancer [55].

The key element in the straightening transform is the algorithm which performs the geometric conversion of outside edges of the examined anatomical structures by rotating contour points in relation to successively identified skeleton points.

The first step in this procedure is to identify the contour points of the object being examined. This process is executed during a single review of the image. A contour point means any point which has at least one direct neighbor belonging to the image background [55]. Once we have identified the edge points and separately established the centerline of the object using a skeletonizing process, we can rotate edge points and thus "straighten" the analyzed organ. In every subsequent step of the algorithm, the rotation process is applied to a pair of points which lie at the intersection of the figure edge with the straight line along which the width of the organ is measured, plotted at the skeleton point being processed at the time. The straight line used to measure the width of the organ is plotted as a straight line running through the skeleton point under consideration, perpendicularly to the guiding line which represents the direction in which the skeleton line runs in this point. The precise method of determining the guiding line (and therefore also the precise description of how to determine the location of the straight line measuring the organ width) are discussed below, but here we can make the intuitive assumption that the measuring straight line is "perpendicular to the skeleton in this point" although it is not very precise to talk about the perpendicularity of a straight line to a curve.

The above operations (plotting a straight line measuring the width of the organ, establishing where it crosses the edge of that organ and performing the appropriate rotation of the identified pair of edge points) are completed subsequently for every skeleton point, and as a result yield a new, straightened contour. The diagram of this procedure is shown in Fig. 5.14.

We will now deal with the details previously omitted. The plotting of guiding lines crossing subsequent skeleton points (the skeleton point currently considered is marked with an A in Figure 5.14) starts from establishing two neighboring (but not directly adjacent!) points which also form part of the skeleton for this skeleton point. Thus, having selected these points, we have a pair of points (marked with B in Figure 5.14) framing the skeleton point A being processed, which framing points are located a specific distance away from it. Such points determine the run of the guiding straight line (shown as C in Figure 5.14). The guiding line helps us to establish the direction of line E, along which the width of the organ is measured (between points shown as F in Figure 5.14).

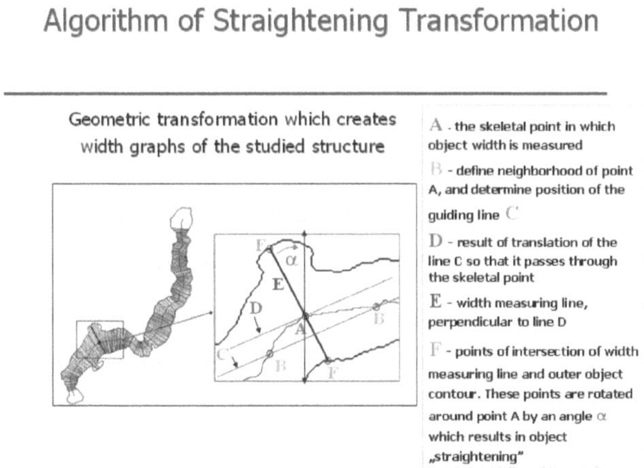

Fig. 5.14. A geometric transform method leading to the determination of the width diagram of the examined structure. Point A stands for the currently analyzed skeleton point in which the object width is established. Point B determines the neighborhood of point A, which allows the directional straight line C to be determined. Straight line D has come into existence as a result of the directional straight line C being translated in such a way that it crosses the current skeleton point A. On the other hand, straight line E is a width measuring straight line, perpendicular to the straight line D. Points F are points at which the width measuring straight line intersects the object's external contour. These points are rotated around point A by angle α (established by straight line E and the OY axis), which leads to 'straightening' the object

Once we have determined the sloping direction of guiding line C intersecting the defined neighborhood of point A, we should translate that straight line so that it would also intersect the skeleton point (A) currently under consideration. This shifted line is labeled D in Figure 5.14.

Determining the width measuring straight line in the currently considered skeleton point is possible thanks to defining the straight line (line E) perpendicular to the previously identified guiding straight line D intersecting the current skeleton point. When the equation of this straight has been determined, it is possible to find the points in which it intersects the object edge, by linearly reviewing all edge points and establishing which of them meet (with the predefined tolerance) the equation representing the width measuring straight line. These points have been labeled F in Figure 5.14. These points may number more than 2, as the structure undergoing examination may have side branches, and one should remember this when viewing the somewhat idealized image of how this procedure runs, shown in Figure 5.14.

Here it is worth going backward a bit to look into a small, but important detail. In the above discussion, we have not explicitly stated what distance should separate points A and B. We will now add that this optimum size of the set neighborhood, as proven by our research, should be approximately equal to the width of the measured object, determined at the previous skeleton point [55]. This allows us to obtain an exceptionally uniform and regular distribution of the width measuring straight lines that are determined.

Now let us come back to the main part of the description of how this method works. Having defined all F points that belong to the edge (contour) of the analyzed anatomical structure and lie along the measurement straight line E, we determine their locations relative to the skeleton, and mainly relative to the previously determined guiding line D in the skeleton point A. To correctly map morphological contour changes to the graph of the object's external edges which is being plotted, it is important to determine the location of these points correctly and precisely.

Geometrically, the most important stage in the straightening transform is the rotation of contour points F determined as described above (they lie along the width measuring straight line E) in relation to the skeleton point A being analyzed, by an α angle equal to the angle by which the width measuring straight line E deviates from the vertical. Such rotations make all width measuring straight lines E vertical, which also causes contour points F determined for all skeleton points A to jointly make up a straightened graph, which shows the external edges of the analyzed object as a shape stretched along a straight line. Such graphs significantly reduce the impact of variable conditions in which the X-rays being used for the diagnosis were taken, and also materially limit distorting factors due to individual variations and the unique shape of the organ being examined belonging to the specific patient. This unified background casts into sharp relief all morphological changes occurring on outside edges of the originally considered anatomical structures and resulting from disease processes under examination (Fig. 5.15).

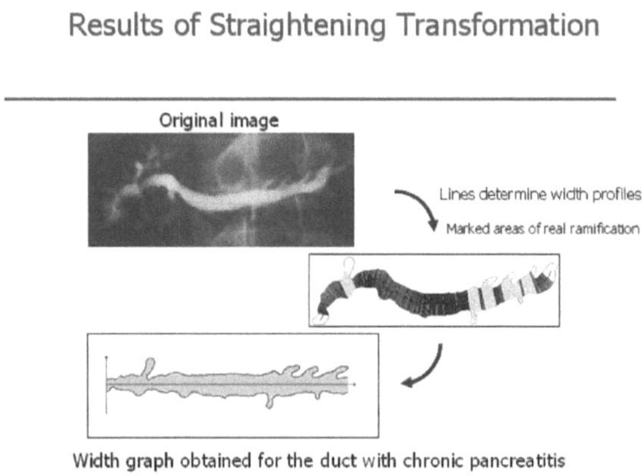

Fig. 5.15. An example of a straightening transform of a pancreatic duct previously subjected to skeletonizing

Our research confirms that this method is very useful in the computer analysis and aiding of automatic medical diagnoses. The utility of the above algorithm has been proven using analyses of various medical images, including ECRP, coronarography images, urograms or spinal cord images [55]. It has been proven that even if the images of organs are very varied both due to the way in which the examination (e.g. the coronarography) was conducted and to very large individual differences, the above algorithm generates 2D graphs of the width of the examined structures which are easy to interpret and which show pathological lesions occurring on the external edges of the examined organs. The type of such lesions and their progress can be identified using various image classification techniques, including pattern comparisons or structural analyses. However, in the context of the main theme of this book, it is important that images thus processed are particularly suitable for generating the semantic description of their structure, which is the key to their automatic understanding.

6. Pattern recognition, clustering and classification applied to selected medical images

6.1. Introduction

The tasks of recognizing images consists in determining that various types of patterns or objects belong to some previously *a priori* defined classes. Recognition can be performed based on rules and principles imposed by an expert who knows that if an image possesses specific characteristics, its specific, precisely defined interpretation is correct. In that case, it is relatively easy to develop a recognition program, as you only need to acquire the image as described in Chapter 2 and possibly process it according to the rules of Chapters 4 and 5, analyze it to distinguish features discussed in Chapter 7, and then it is sufficient to use an algorithm which represents the expert's opinion in a language understandable to a computer in order to classify the objects. The above situation sometimes occurs in medicine, as for many diseases there are strict standards which allow one to tell an image acquired of a healthy patient apart from an image indicating the presence of some pathologies. However, such a recognition based on applying rules can only be used for relatively simple problems. In the case of many other jobs, responding to specific medical needs, we find that there is no a priori information about the rules of these or those objects (and their images) belonging to specific pattern classes. In that situation, the only information that the classifying algorithm can use is that contained in the so-called training set, i.e. a sequence of patterns comprising objects for which the correct classification is known [18, 26]. The need to refer to a training set makes the job of image recognition extremely interesting as an example of a problem which requires the computer to conduct inductive reasoning.

We know that even a rather slow person can solve a problem if he/she is given a general rule for proceeding. This method of problem solving is called the deduction method. Computers can also do this, as every computer program is really a form of such a deductive rule. However, real intelligence (natural or artificial) is expressed in the ability to independently discover an unknown rule for proceeding in a situation where the only known information comprises examples of that rule's operation. Consequently, image recognition problems have always represented one of the most typical jobs for artificial intelligence, precisely because there are no defined rules for the recognition algorithm. In practice, this means that a computer recognizing images must to some extent learn to recognize new patterns on the basis of examples presented to it before. Fortunately, in the medical image recognition field considered here, it is relatively easy to accumulate the necessary set of examples, as there is no problem to collect from clinical archives large numbers of medical images together with the diagnoses verified by completed therapies and their results.

M.R. Ogiela and R. Tadeusiewicz: *Pattern recognition, clustering and classification applied to selected medical images,* Studies in Computational Intelligence (SCI) **84**, 117–151 (2007)
www.springerlink.com

A crucial element in training image recognition algorithms is their generalization, which means that the algorithm can not only accumulate knowledge based on the patterns provided to it, but after completing the learning can also classify completely new images which did not form part of the training sequence: and thus it can be used in practice to diagnose subsequent patients.

Relatively simple images showing repetitive objects with little individual variation (e.g. printed characters) can be recognized based on a simple analysis of the image as such, e.g. by comparing it to a stored pattern. However, in the case of many medical image classes, the varied nature of objects that may constitute the objects to be recognized necessitates a recognition process whose preliminary stage is to detect the characteristic features of specific patterns. In this kind of recognition, the next step consists in analyzing the detected features and ends in an attempt to make a decision, i.e. to classify the image. The subject of features which can be used to analyze and recognize medical images has been discussed separately in Chapter 7, so we will not be returning to it here, but we should emphasize that in recognition, the most important features of the image are those that can be called its distinctive features.

To summarize the above discussion we can say that the image recognition job is most frequently connected with a multi-stage process of information processing during which the quantity of analyzed data is greatly reduced. Information in the form of an image can take huge volumes of computer storage, because a medical image is recorded at a high spatial and amplitude resolution and can use as much as several gigabytes. The image is processed during its analysis. As a result, the same contents telling one what is visible in the image and what it means can be expressed using less data in the form of a vector of features used for various purposes, including the recognition. The latter also further reduces information quantity, since automatic classification assigns the number of one of the recognized classes to the object, and that number can then replace a long vector of analyzed features which requires great precision of representation.

Before we go into detailed considerations on the automatic recognition of medical images, let us also review the problem more globally, starting from historical assumptions and pre-classifying the methods to be considered.

Image recognition methods date back to the pioneering period in the development of artificial intelligence methods which took place in 1950s. The first practical implementations of image recognition techniques were based on neural network systems developed by Rosenblatt in 1968, generally known under the name of Perceptron. These systems were based on a structure of several layers built of electronic artificial neurons, which contained the calculation data, the recognition-facilitating premises accumulated during the learning process, and the output arrays which took the final decisions.

These first experiments in artificial intelligence and image recognition produced two important conclusions, which accelerated subsequent research:

1. Hardware's ability to learn is an indispensable attribute of machine intelligence; and

2. Human intelligence consists in 99% of image (pattern) recognition, and only in 1% of the reasoning itself [52].

That second statement, albeit questioned by some scientists, strongly accelerated research on automatic image recognition, as apart from people who wanted to solve specific problems (like character recognition or fingerprint identification), quite a number interested in the foundations of artificial intelligence also got involved in the recognition field. Consequently, a number of methods for automatic image recognition were developed and analyzed, many of which are still successfully used today. The first to appear were classical image recognition methods based on minimum distance techniques. Their forefather was the nearest neighbor method (NN) [18, 52, 54], which will be described further down in this chapter. That method was notionally easy, but relatively failure-prone, so modifications of it were developed, i.e. algorithms insensitive to errors in the training sequence, such as the αNN or the j_NNN methods. Even though these methods were the forefathers of all other image recognition methods, they are still frequently used today, as they exhibit a high precision of object recognition, even at the price of major requirements for memory use and calculation time.

Subsequent classical methods of image recognition, which appeared alongside minimum distance ones, were the approximation and probabilistic methods. These will also be characterized in greater detail further down in this chapter. They represent a completely different way of developing the object classification algorithm, but in many cases yield similar results and a similar effectiveness of recognition to those achieved by minimum distance methods, but with much smaller load on the recognizing system, both in terms of memory use and calculation time.

As mentioned above, the above methods successfully solved many practical problems, like automatic barcode reading at shops, OCR, coin identification by vending machines (selling beverages, for instance), recognizing simple spoken commands etc. These methods (in particular those based on probabilistic schemes) have been successfully applied in medicine, although not for medical image recognition, but to aid the diagnostic process conducted based on numerical (biochemical analysis results) or descriptive data (results of medical history taking).

With regard to the increasingly important medical data in the form of images acquired by various types of imaging equipment (e.g. CT or USG), classical image recognition methods are generally ineffective, particularly when recognizing patterns composed of many objects. This problem was solved by the development of syntactic methods using mathematical linguistics methods, called syntactic image recognition methods [18, 55].

1980s saw a boom in research on neural networks and the possibility of using them for pattern classification jobs. At that time, several effective, formal and heuristic methods of multi-layer network learning were proposed [26], which enabled pattern recognition based on following examples from the so-called training set, then properly generalized into patterns not shown during the learning, but characterized by a specific level of similarity to the former. However, neural networks are of only limited utility to analyze and classify complex medical images, since the image as such (particularly a high resolution one) cannot be input into the neural network, and the attempts to teach networks to recognize images based on their features extracted by preprocessing have not yielded any significant advantage over techniques based on the above minimum distance, approximation or probabilistic methods.

Due to the development of all these methods, we now have many varied ways of identifying different kinds of patterns and of automatically classifying images (including medical ones). The number of image recognition methods currently known is large and keeps rising, as many authors, particularly of doctors' theses, ambitiously keep making new attempts to develop novel methods and algorithms. This shows how very current and very attractive automatic classification and computer recognition still are as a scientific field. However, the huge number of these methods also proves that none of them is completely and definitely good, because if one best method had been developed and then indisputably proven to be advantageous over other methods in numerous research projects, everyone would want to use only that method and would forego all others. However, those numerous recognition methods exist, and over all these years they were developed and perfected so that they would successfully recognize even very complex images and patterns. Examples of such applications will be presented in further sections of this chapter.

Figure 6.1 presents the general classification of image recognition methods.

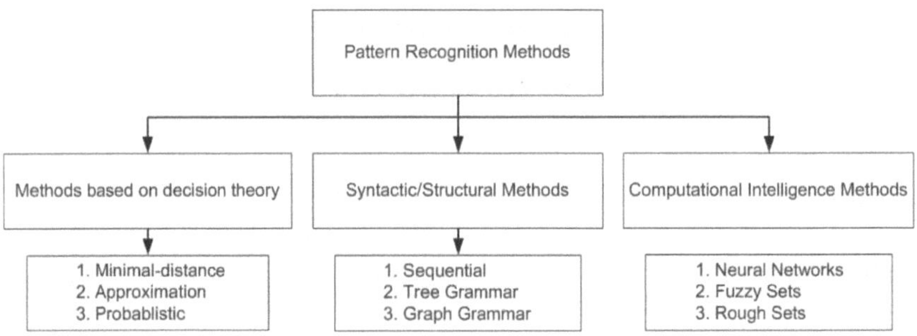

Fig. 6.1. The general classification of image recognition methods

Subsequent chapters will characterize techniques selected from among these methods in greater detail. In particular, we will enlarge on methods based on computational intelligence, which include neural networks, methods based on the decision-making theory and syntactic methods using image languages.

6.2. A general model of medical image recognition

The purpose of an image recognition job is to construct an algorithm capable of classifying analyzed patterns based on some characteristics distinguished in the image [54]. In mathematical terms, such an algorithm can be written as the following mapping:

$$A : D \rightarrow I \cup \{i_0\}, \text{ where:}$$

- D – a set of objects to be recognized
- I – defines the set of classes of objects being recognized
- i_0 – means the neutral identification, meaning the lack of a decision (very important!)

In particular, mapping A is executed as the composition of three recognition stages set in the form of subsequent mappings:

$$A = F \bullet C \bullet B, \text{ where:}$$

- B – a function of pattern reception
- C – a function of pattern-describing vectors belonging to particular classes;
- F – a decision-making (classification) function which facilitates an unanimous assignation to a recognized class or generates the message that such a classification cannot be made.

The first stage in recognizing any objects is to measure the significant features of objects undergoing recognition. This measurement defines the perception function set in the following form:

$$B: D \rightarrow X, \text{ where X is the space of features.}$$

The notion of a feature is of particular importance here. In general it refers to the property of the pattern being recognized (e.g. an image) which can be expressed in a quantitative or a qualitative form, and which differentiates the objects being recognized well.

The ability to define significant features allows the objects being recognized $d \in D$ to be replaced with n-dimensional points in the feature space X. The elements of this space are n-element vectors $\underline{x} = (x_1, x_2, \ldots x_n) \in X$ which describe major parameters of the recognized objects.

According to the Brawermann principle [54], features which form the components of such vectors shall be selected so that the points corresponding to objects belonging to one class should make up groups in the feature space X which groups are well separated from similar groups forming for other classes [18].

Having defined the feature vector, the next stage in the recognition process is to establish whether an unknown object $d \in D$ belongs to individual classes. The process consists in calculating the values of belonging functions to all the classes considered. This stage of the recognition process is defined by the following mapping:

$$C: X \rightarrow \mathcal{R}^L$$

where $\mathcal{R}$ – denotes the set of real numbers and L – the number of classes being recognized.

In order to perform such a mapping, we use the defined feature vector $\underline{x}$ (determined by the perception function) to calculate the values of the belonging function for every pattern being recognized in turn. Values of these functions define the measure of the belonging of the unknown object d to particular classes, so they are real numbers (usually positive). As the quantity of these numbers which has to be determined is equal to the quantity of classes under consideration, transform C yields the set L of such numbers, which is formally written as an element of an L-dimensional space of real numbers $\mathcal{R}^L$.

The final stage in image recognition is to take the final decision that the correct recognition has been made (or that it is impossible to achieve a recognition) using the following mapping:

$$F: \mathcal{R}^L \rightarrow I \cup \{i_0\}$$

According to the classification function F, a decision is made that the object $d \in D$, (described at this time by the feature vector $\underline{x} \in D$) belongs to that class $i \in I$ for which the value of the appropriate belonging function is the highest. Details of all these stages are described in book [54]. The most simplified diagram of the recognition process is presented in Figure 6.2.

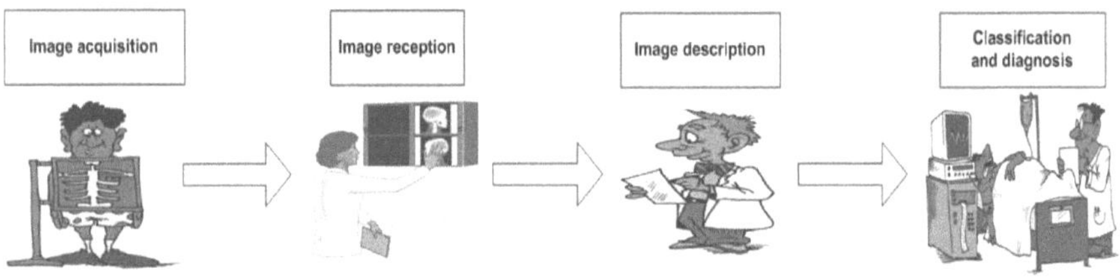

Fig. 6.2. Stages in recognizing medical images

6.3. Clustering as a symmetrical problem for classification and pattern recognition

Clustering is a process similar to pattern classification, but in a sense going in the opposite direction. In the recognition job described above we first had set classes, and then for specific data we had to indicate which class they fitted best. In clustering, we first have data, and then we look for classes that fit that data best. In this case, the process is mainly aimed at grouping data according to some features or a key. In clustering, the data examples provided and the entire training sequence have no identification labels that would allow that data to be assigned to some patterns. However, this technique does not consist in the simple grouping of data, but also in discovering (as a result of the learning process) and delivering for the subsequent use of a certain set of rules or mathematical equations to differentiate such groups.

A clustering job is best illustrated with the simple example from Figure 6.3. Let us assume two features describing a person: their height and weight. Using these features, data can be presented in a 2D coordinate system.

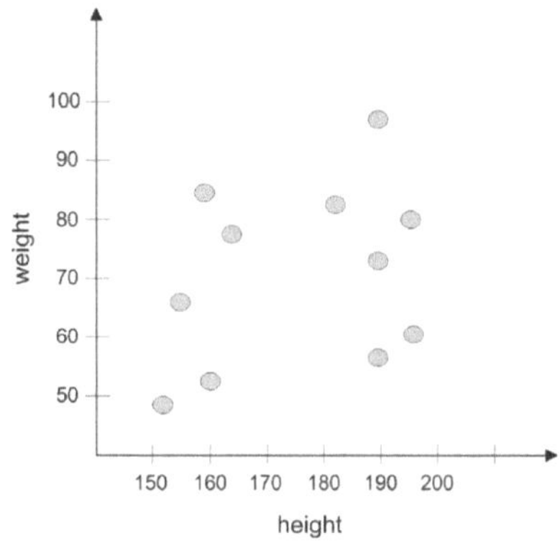

Fig. 6.3. A 2D feature space representing the weight and height of a group of people

In this example we can observe that the points it shows can be assigned to four groups of people defined as follows:

- Group 1 – Short people (<175) of low weight (< 70)
- Group 2 – Short people (<175) of high weight (>70)
- Group 3 – Tall people (>175) of medium weight (>70 and < 90)
- Group 4 – Tall people (>175) of high weight (>90)

Taking into account the criterion of health standards of people representing particular groups you can also observe that in theory people from groups 1 and 4 should be more healthy (because they keep the right proportion of body weight to height) than those from the remaining two groups. It is easy to see that by introducing the above breakdown we have solved the clustering problem of establishing some characteristic subgroups for the group of people under consideration. The clustering introduced above was, however, rather a result of the scientist's own thinking and was done somewhat "manually". From the point of view of the purposes and jobs considered in this book, more important and useful are clustering methods that allow natural groups of the considered data and the requisite decision-making rules to be automatically defined.

One of the simplest automatic clustering methods is the k-means method, which represents one of the most popular techniques applied, among other purposes, to medical image analysis. This method assumes that there are k groups of patterns characteristic for the data in question, and the clustering algorithm tries to find optimum groups in the feature space and the location of patterns for particular classes.

This is how that method works:

For n input samples (x_o, x_1, ..., x_{n-1}), the k-means method is used to develop k clusters, whereas for each one of them, a nodal element is determined which represents the conventional mean of the entire group in the feature space. The k-means method operates by iterations. In order to find the best locations for mean points of every cluster, it first takes random locations, and then improves them so as to best adjust every pattern to the input data cluster whose centre is the closest to the pattern.

In the k-means method, learning can be described in the following steps:

1. Defining the mean points of particular classes using original values $m_0, m_1, \ldots, m_{k-1}$. At the beginning, those are vectors randomly spread in the space of input signals.
2. Determining the distances between all samples $(x_o, x_1, \ldots, x_{n-1})$ in the sequence and all the mean points of classes $m_0, m_1, \ldots, m_{k-1}$,
3. $d_{ij}(x_i, m_j) = \| x_i - m_j \| = \left((x_{i1} - m_{j1})^2 + \ldots + (x_{ip} - m_{jp})^2 \right)^{\frac{1}{2}}$, for $i = 0,\ldots,n-1$ and $j = 0,\ldots, k-1$
4. Combining into one group all those input signals x_i from among the samples $(x_o, x_1, \ldots, x_{n-1})$ whose distance to the mean point m_j of class j is shorter than the distance of the same input signals x_i to the mean points m_l of other classes ($l \neq j$), in order to create class j. This action is performed for all numbers of classes $j = 0,\ldots, k-1$.
5. Finding new mean points of classes by looking among signals x_i for the sample whose coordinates are the closest to the mean values of coordinates determined for all input signals which have been allocated to class j. (In a variety of this method which allows the class pattern to be an abstract object that does not belong to the set of samples $x_o, x_1, \ldots, x_{n-1}$, the mean point of class j is simply a point whose coordinates are the means of coordinates of elements x_i assigned to that class.)
6. If during the last iteration no element x_i changed its class, the clustering process should be terminated, if not, go back to (3).
7. Process ends. The finally formed clusters and their means $m_0, m_1, \ldots, m_{k-1}$ form the output values of the algorithm.

To illustrate this process, we can analyze the following example (Fig. 6.4).

If we assume the number of clusters searched for as K = 3, step 1 should activate the mean points of three clusters.

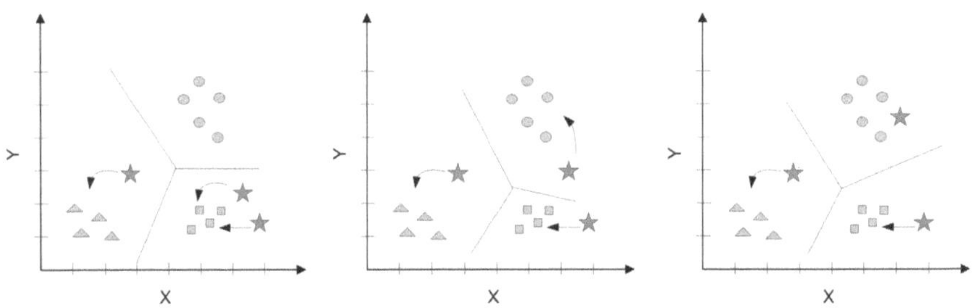

Fig. 6.4. A) Activating cluster mean points, B) Effects of assigning mean points to cluster, C) Final selection of new mean points of clusters

Figure 6.4.A presents the activation of initial mean points. It shows that the mean points of clusters for “square” and “round” patterns in reality may belong to the same cluster. In the next step, for every pattern present in the feature space, the right cluster of input data belonging to that pattern should be determined. This selection is made according to the distance between the patterns and cluster mean points. Figure 6.4.B shows the effect of such an assignment. Then we have to determine the **means** of elements in each output cluster to find new mean points of those clusters. Usually this process shifts the mean values of the clusters under consideration closer to the actual centers of gravity of the naturally appearing groups of data under consideration.

In every subsequent iteration, the process of determining the mean points and grouping elements from feature space around them is repeated using data obtained during the previous iteration. As a result, the mean points determined migrate (which can be observed in the feature space) towards the centers of gravity of particular natural groupings of input data.

When repeating the iteration no longer yields changes in the location of patterns and the belonging of input data to clusters, the cluster mean points are assumed to have been finally selected (Figure 6.4.C).

The k-means method described above is the most popular, but by no means the only method of automatic clustering.

In the classification of medical patterns, fuzzy clustering is also frequently used. These methods are particularly useful if the distributions of the probability density function for every class are not precisely known or when the clusters themselves do not exhibit compact shapes in the feature space. In such cases, fuzzy clustering is used, as it allows the input vectors to belong to more than one cluster at the same time.

6.4. Simple pattern recognition methods (e.g. the k-neighbors algorithm and similar metrics-based methods) in medical applications

This chapter presents minimum distance methods in which the *C* mapping (measuring the degree to which specific data belongs to individual classes) is linked to the notion of **distance** in feature space *X*. This space must therefore be furnished with the appropriate **metric.** The metric can consist in any mapping that fulfills the following axioms.

For all vectors $x^{\mu} \in X$ ($\mu = 1, 2, \ldots$) the metric meets the following assumptions:

$$\rho(\underline{x}^{\mu}, \underline{x}^{v}) = 0 \Leftarrow \underline{x}^{\mu} \equiv \underline{x}^{v},$$

$$\rho(\underline{x}^{\mu}, \underline{x}^{v}) = \rho(\underline{x}^{v}, \underline{x}^{\mu}),$$

$$\rho(\underline{x}^{\mu}, \underline{x}^{v}) < \rho(\underline{x}^{\mu}, \underline{x}^{n}) + \rho(\underline{x}^{n}, \underline{x}^{v}).$$

As mappings that meet such conditions are potentially infinite in number, so the author of the recognition method enjoys a lot of freedom in how to define and use the appropriate metric. However, it should be noted that in practical applications of minimum distance methods the effectiveness of a given method is frequently very highly dependent on the selected metric, which has a major influence on the results achieved [18, 54].

In minimum distance methods, the idea behind identifying and classifying unknown patterns consists in selecting, as the appropriate identification, the number of the class $i \in I$ which contains the pattern $\underline{x}^{i,k}$ closest (according to the adopted metric) to the object d being recognized (represented by feature vector $\underline{x}$).

Minimum distance methods are based on premises relating to the geometry of the feature space. So if the points that correspond to objects of different classes gather into clear concentrations (as in Figure 6.4, for example), then it is productive to use values of distance (measured using the metric introduced) when taking the decision to classify the new pattern.

NN method (nearest neighbor)

One of the simplest minimum distance methods is the NN (nearest neighbor) method. The decision-making rule in the NN algorithm says that an unknown object will be classified to the class to which the object of the training sequence closest in the feature space to the unknown one belongs (Figure 6.5).

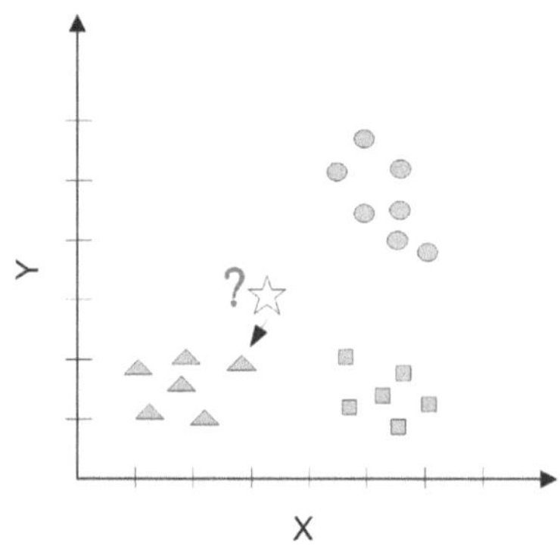

Fig. 6.5. Examples of pattern groups in the feature space and the method of classifying a new element

The NN method is frequently used in medical diagnostics applications, as it is notionally simple and corresponds to the intuitively acceptable principle of indicating (as a probable diagnosis) the illness suffered by the patient whose symptoms are the most similar to those displayed by the patient currently examined.

k-NN method (k-nearest neighbors)

As the classical NN method is very sensitive to errors in the training sequence, then if even a single element from the training sequence is determined to belong to the wrong group, its entire neighborhood will be incorrectly classified and assigned to the same group as the incorrectly determined element from the training sequence (Figure 6.6.A).

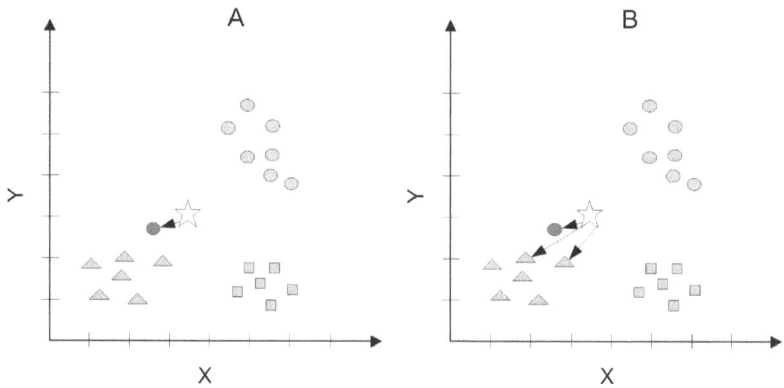

Fig. 6.6. The k-NN method (here k = 3) prevents errors resulting from mistakes in the training sequence (A) and yields correct classifications (B).

To minimize the number of wrong classifications, methods are introduced in which the decision is taken on the basis of more objects from the training sequence located closest to the object of unknown classification, an these objects vote in a way. If one assumes that the number of voting objects is *k,* then the relevant method is called k-NN. In this method *k* is used as a parameter whose choice determines properties of the method. This parameter is selected arbitrarily, as a small natural number, smaller than the number of elements in the smallest of the recognized classes.

In this method, the classification process is performed in such a way that after the *k* value is determined for the recognized pattern $\underline{x}$, values of its distance from all elements of the training sequence are calculated, i.e. the distances $\rho(\underline{x}, \underline{x}^k)$ are determined for $k = 1,2.....,$ N. Then we order the training sequence in line with the increasing distance from the pattern recognized, and a new numbering of $v = 1,$ 2..., n is introduced for the sequence thus sorted. The sorted training sequence is therefore defined as:

$$U = \{\langle \underline{x}^{v}, i^{v} \rangle, v = 1,2....,N\},$$

whereas

$$\forall_{v,\mu}[v > \mu \Rightarrow \rho(\underline{x}, \underline{x}^v) > \rho(\underline{x}, \underline{x}^\mu)$$

Then we select *k* initial objects of that training sequence and create the subset

$$U^{\alpha} = \{\langle \underline{x}^{v}, i^{v} \rangle,\ v = 1, 2, \ldots.., \alpha\}$$

which is split into subsets (frequently empty) associated with particular classes

$$U^{\alpha,i} = \{\langle \underline{x}^{v}, i^{v} \rangle,\ v < \alpha \cap i^{v} = i\}$$

Functions of belonging for the *k-NN* method can now be determined on the basis of the size of particular subsets $U^{\alpha,i}$

$$C^{i}(\underline{x}) = \# U^{\alpha,i};\ i = 1, 2\ldots.., L$$

Finally, the new pattern is classified to the class which has the most numerous representation among the k elements nearest to that pattern in the entire training sequence.

The algorithm j_N-*NN* exhibits properties related to the *k-NN* presented here. The essence of this algorithm is to determine that an unknown object belongs to the class to which the j_N^{th} subsequent element of the training subset U ordered in accordance with the rules described for *k-NN* belongs to. Usually, this modification can be written in the form of the following belonging function:

$$C^i(\underline{x}) = \delta_{ijNi},$$

where the compliance function δ is determined by the Kronecker delta function.

When characterizing minimum distance algorithms we can say that they are frequently applied in practice due to their simplicity and intuitive nature, and also due to their high effectiveness. However, their drawback is the high computational and memory complexity. These methods require the entire training sequence to be allocated in the memory of the recognizing computer and require calculating the distance ρ between the object being recognized and all elements of the training sequence; they also require the time-consuming sorting of these elements to select *k* nearest neighbors.

6.5. Pattern recognition methods based on approximating regions in feature space

This section describes approximation methods. In these methods, the function of pattern belonging to particular classes $C^i(\underline{x})$ is expanded into a series in relation to a defined family of base functions φ

$$\forall i \in I \left[\forall \underline{x} \in X \left[C^i(\underline{x}) = \sum_{v=0}^{\infty} V_v^i \varphi_v(\underline{x}) \right] \right]$$

where the base functions used form an ordered family

$$\Phi = \left\langle \varphi_1(\underline{x}), \varphi_2(\underline{x}), \ldots \right\rangle$$

Coefficients of this expansion, i.e. the values V_v^i, act as "weights" that allow us to determine a specific function $C^i(\underline{x})$. These coefficients are material in the sense that for a set family of functions Φ, the problem of determining decision-making rules for particular classes is replaced by the problem of determining the values of weights V_v^i. For the process of weight value establishing to be effectively conducted by the computer, we need to restrict the range of summation in the formula which defines the extension of the belonging function, as an infinite scope of summation, just as an infinite set of weights, obviously cannot be used in practice. As a result of such a simplification, the formula takes the following form:

$$C^i(\underline{x}) = \sum_{v=0}^{m} V_v^i \varphi_v(\underline{x})$$

This form implies a very favorable situation, as in order to determine all belonging functions we only need to determine $L*m$ of coefficients V^i_v, which are also the only information to be remembered during further recognition. In contrast to the need to store the entire training sequence U for minimum distance methods, this is a major simplification. The problem of selecting base functions has been discussed broadly in [54].

6.5.1. Linear approximation of boundaries between regions

When we have a defined a family of functions Φ, then based on the training sequence U we can determine the weight coefficients V^i_η of the expansions of the belonging functions. These functions, at special assumptions that $m = n$ and $\varphi_v(\underline{x}) = x_v$ (where $\varphi_0(\underline{x}) \equiv 1$ out of the definition), allow us to obtain expansions of the belonging function in the form of the following linear function:

$$C^i(\underline{x}) = \sum_{v=1}^{\eta} V_\eta^i x_v + V_0^i$$

Once we have this form of the function, we can easily derive the rules of iterative determination of weight coefficients V^i, as these can be established precisely on the basis of a reasoning according to which the process of selecting weight coefficients V^i is the result of gradient optimization aimed at minimizing the error committed by the automatic classifier. The details of this derivation are presented in publication [54]. The formula quoted above, together with the appropriate method of learning weight coefficients V^i, jointly define the recognition rule that can be used as the optimum function of belonging to classes which are linearly separated in the feature space.

In practice, we are never certain whether the problem under consideration (the classes) is linearly separable (Figure 6.7), so it makes sense to attempt to use this method as the first in a row (because if its works, then we obtain a convenient classifier without additional complications), but we have to be ready for the need to precisely verify the result and to change the belonging functions into a non-linear function if the classifier generates too many errors.

The use of linear belonging functions has the following advantages:

1. The recognition algorithm is simple, and the belonging function itself is easy to calculate
2. The number of elements that need to be stored is very small: it is enough to store $L(n + 1)$ weight coefficients V^i_v

3. The learning algorithm is easy to execute and boils down to determining the value of V^i based on sequence U.

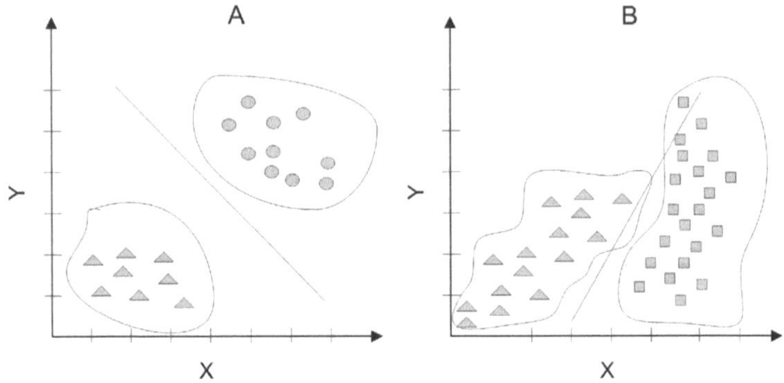

Fig. 6.7. Two classes in the feature space. A) linearly separated, B) classes linearly non-separable. If the objects of linearly non-separable classes are split by a hyperplane, even one selected very carefully, wrong recognitions will appear

One interesting aspect of this method is that the formula defining the belonging function can also be interpreted as the simplest description of the neuron function. Here, the human ability to recognize objects has become a kind of pattern for recognition jobs considered in practice. This subject will be expanded on in the further sections dealing with neural networks.

The way of learning and determining weights in recognizing with the linear function method has been described at length in [54].

6.5.2. SVM: a simple and effective method of pattern recognition

The SVM (Support Vector Machines-) technique consists in preprocessing data in such a way that patterns can be presented using feature vectors of a high dimension, usually much greater than the originally considered feature space. By using the appropriate non-linear mapping which allows us to achieve a sufficiently high dimension, all data (e.g. from two categories, but not separable linearly in the original feature space) can always be divided by the appropriate hyperplane in a space of the appropriately higher dimensionality.

Let us therefore assume that every pattern x_k will be transformed into a new, extended form using the function $y_k = \varphi(x_k)$. For every one of the n patterns considered ($k=1, 2, ..., n$), let the value $z_k=\pm 1$ be set, depending on whether the pattern k is in class ω_1 or in class ω_2. In the extended space y, the linear discriminant will have the form $g(y) = a^t y$, where the weight vector a and the transformed vector of pattern y are extended by $a_0 = w_0$ and $y_0=1$, respectively. This is why the hyperplane which originally splits the classes, after it is introduced, ensures their linear cohesion (which means that all data is on the same side of the transformed hyperplane):

$$z_k g(y_k) \geq 1, k = 1, \ldots, n$$

The purpose of training the SVM is to find such a hyperplane separating the classes which has the greatest margins that still allow the patterns to be classified correctly. It is assumed that the greater the margin, the better the generalization of the classifier. The distance between any hyperplane and the transformed pattern y is set in the form of $|g(y)|/||a||$. Consequently, if a positive margin b exists, the following estimation is true:

$$\frac{z_k g(y_k)}{\| a \|} \geq b, \text{ dla } k = 1, \ldots, n$$

For this formula, the purpose is to find a weight vector a which maximizes value b. As the target vector may be changed arbitrarily and still determine the correct hyperplane, the limitation $b||a|| = 1$ is imposed. The solution considered to be correct should also minimize the value $||a||^2$.

Support vectors are transformed patterns for which the above formula is fulfilled in the limiting way, i.e. there is an equality instead of inequality. Patterns are then equidistant from the hyperplane generated and are treated as training samples which define the optimum separation of the hyperplane dividing particular classes. Such patterns are the most useful in the classification process, as they provide the most information (Figure 6.8).

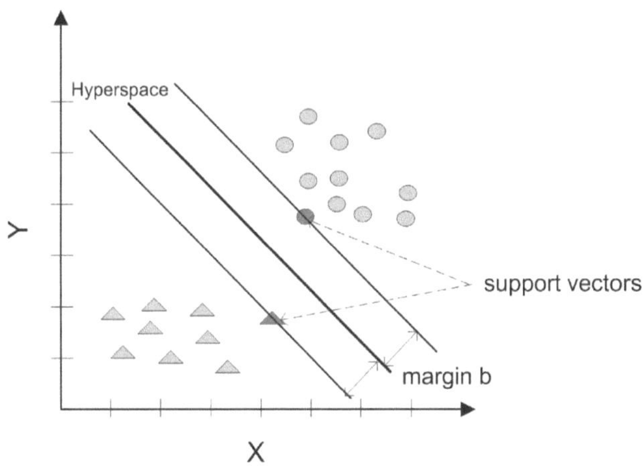

Fig. 6.8. Support vectors lie on lines marking the margins. The separating hyperplane is drawn in the centre

To train an SVM, the first step is to select nonlinear functions which will transform input patterns into a space of a new (higher) dimension. This is frequently imposed top down, but if this information is missing, we can use the Gauss function or any other family of well parameterized functions. The dimensionality of the space being transformed can be of any height, but is usually restricted by the computational capacity. To minimize the value of the weight vector, the following formula is used:

$$L(a,\alpha) = \frac{1}{2} \| a \|^2 - \sum_{k=1}^{n} \alpha_k \left[z_k a^t y_k - 1 \right]$$

We should minimize the value of L in relation to the weight vector a and maximize it in relation to multipliers $\alpha_k \geq 0$.

6.5.3. Nonlinear methods and nonlinear transformations in region modeling

The method of linear functions described in previous sections was based on using the linear approximation of the expansion of a belonging function into a finite series of base functions. However, it may sometimes turn out that such expansions for the belonging function will not allow us to obtain satisfactory recognition results (as shown in Fig. 6.7.B). However, it so happens that in special cases an expansion formula set in that way allows dividing planes of any shape to be defined, and not just in the shape of hyperplanes as in the case of linear approximations. For example, the use of second degree polynomials as base functions makes it possible to obtain ellipsoids, paraboloids, hyperboloids and any combinations of them as the separating structures. It also turns out that the effectiveness of recognition (of separating classes in the feature space) is influenced by the number of selectable coefficients m, which are available in the expansion of belonging functions. There is a theorem about the relationship between the number of weights determined and the probability of a correct recognition [26]. This theorem shows that if we increase m in case of problems with recognition, we get better results. Consequently, it is reasonable to select a recognition method based on the belonging function with the following general form:

$$C^i(\underline{x}) = \sum_{v=0}^{m} V_v^i \varphi_v(\underline{x})$$

For such a function, the learning process (consisting in finding weights V_v^i) is conducted similarly as for linear functions, with the difference that we set a transformation of the n-dimensional feature space into a “straightening” m-dimensional space in which the areas belonging to different classes not linearly paired in the feature space can be separated with hyperplanes. The details of this operation are described in [54].

It has already been mentioned that the probability of making the correct identification clearly rises if we use nonlinear functions instead of linear ones, and if the length of the expansion of the belonging function is based on a greater number of base functions than the considered number of object classes, i.e. $m >> n$.

For example, for the square belonging function, $C^i(\underline{x})$ the length of the expansion can be determined using the following formula: $m = n(n + 3)/2$.

For a belonging function $C^i(\underline{x})$ which generally represents a μ-degree polynomial, the length of its expansion into a series can be:

$$m = \binom{n+\mu}{\mu} - 1, \text{ where } \binom{n+\mu}{\mu} = \frac{(n+\mu)!}{n!\,\mu!} \text{ denotes the Newton symbol.}$$

The impact of the value of m on the probability of the correct identification can be estimated as below.

As N points (e.g. all the elements of the training sequence) can be split into 2 classes (for the simplest case of L = 2) in the total of 2^N ways assuming that no three points lie along the same straight line, then in an m-dimensional space, these N points can be split with hyperplanes in $L(N, m)$ ways. This shows that the probability of recreating the necessary assignment of N points to 2 classes using the division generated in the process of linear learning can be estimated using the following formula:

$$prob(N, m) = \frac{L(N,m)}{2^N}$$

To justify the phenomenon that the increase of m raises the probability of the correct identification, it is enough to prove that $prob(N, m)$ is a growing function of its second argument. Any $L(N, m)$ values can be calculated from the recurrent formula:

$$L(N,m) = L(N-1,m) + L(N-1,m-1)$$

used with the obvious limiting conditions:

$$L(1,m) = 2 \text{ and } L(N,1) = 2N$$

To make calculations easier, the variability of this function is better presented in a table.

Table 6.1 summarizes the values of $L(N, m)$ for $N < 8$ and $m < 6$

Table 6.1. Values of function $L(N, m)$) source [54]

Value of N	Dimension of the feature space m				
	1	2	3	4	5
1	2	2	2	2	2
2	4	4	4	4	4
3	6	8	8	8	8
4	8	14	16	16	16
5	10	22	30	32	32
6	12	32	52	62	64
7	14	44	84	114	126
8	16	58	128	198	240

Knowing the values $L(N, m)$ we can determine the shape of the probability $prob(N, m)$. In this case $\lim_{m \to 0} prob(N,m) = 0$ and $\lim_{m \to \infty} prob(N,m) = 1$.

From the practical application standpoint, however, it will be easier to state that $prob(N, m^*) = 1/2$ for the critical value of $m^* = \frac{1}{2}N - 1$ and to note that around m^* there is a quick transition from $prob(N,m) = 0$ to $prob(N, m) = 1$.

This unanimously proves that as the dimension of the space m increases, the probability of the correct identification also rises. However, we should remember that m should rise in such a way as to introduce components which really contribute new information. Those may be additional features x_i, but they may also be new transformations φ_v of features $\underline{x}$ already recorded.

6.6. Neural networks for medical image recognition

Neural networks are systems of interconnected neurons which process information in parallel. To a limited extent such neurons model the operation of real, biological neurons which make up structures responsible for image perception and recognition as well as the interpretation of all other signals and stimuli in the brain. Neurons are composed of a part with multiple inputs called synapses and the output part called the axon.

Properties of particular neurons are determined by weight coefficients of synapses $V^{(\lambda)}{}_v$ (also called synaptic weights) which identify every input number v of every cell in network number λ, and by the additional coefficient $V_0^{(\lambda)}$ referred to as the neural threshold or the BIAS.

The advantage of neural networks stems from the way they operate: by processing data in parallel, and their ability to learn on the basis of the input data they are fed. They can be used to execute specific jobs by correctly controlling the connections between neurons and by specifying synaptic weights. The process of weight determination consists in training the network and for every network type there is an algorithm which allows that network to be trained in such a way as to achieve its desirable properties. Learning algorithms can be split into two types. There are algorithms for supervised learning and for unsupervised learning. For supervised learning, the input data and correct results, called training samples, are fed to the network. The process is conducted by directly comparing the output data to the correct solutions previously fed to the network. Unsupervised learning occurs if the input data fed in lacks patterns or correct results used to determine which solution is correct.

In order to determine the processes occurring in a single network node (neuron), the value of the aggregate stimulation of the neuron during the presentation of the kth element of the training sequence:

$$\tilde{e}_{\lambda}^{k} = \sum_{\nu=1}^{n} V_{\nu}^{(\lambda)(k-1)} x_{\nu}^{k} + V_{0}^{(\lambda)}$$

is linked to its output signal with some non-linear function

$$\tilde{x}_{\lambda}^{k} = \varphi\left[\tilde{e}_{\lambda}^{k}\right]$$

A neural network usually has a layered structure. It can be divided into the input layer which receives input signals from the outside and the output layer whose signals may indicate the output value.

If the component x_ν of the feature vector $\underline{x}$ is the external input to the νth input of every neuron of the first layer, and $\tilde{x}_{\lambda}$ is the output signal from the λth neuron of the network, then the learning process will consist of presenting k patterns from the training sequence U to the network in subsequent steps and assessing the output signals generated by that network,

$$W = \left\{\tilde{x}_{\lambda}^{k}, k = 1,2,\dots,N; \lambda \in \mathrm{N}\right\}$$

compared to the pattern for which the network is to aim

$$Z = \left\{\hat{x}_{\lambda}^{k}, k = 1,2,\dots,N; \lambda \in \mathrm{N}\right\}$$

Coefficients $V^{(\lambda)}_{\nu}$ change during the presentation of signals $\tilde{x}_{\nu}^{k}$ by a value $\Delta V_{\nu}^{(\lambda)(k)}$, whereas the learning rule is expressed by the following formula:

$$\Delta V_{\nu}^{(\lambda)(k)} = \varsigma_1 \left(\hat{x}_{\lambda}^{k} - \tilde{x}_{\lambda}^{k}\right) \frac{d\varphi^{k}}{d\tilde{e}_{\lambda}} x_{\nu}^{k}$$

The characteristics of neural networks have led to their very successful application to solve various problems of identifying and classifying medical images [52].

Three basic types of neural networks are distinguished:

1. Recurrent (Hopfield) nets. These are nonlinear networks with a generalized feedback scheme in which neurons are interconnected so that the output of every one of them is sent (as a feedback signal) to the inputs of all the others. These networks have various applications, but are most frequently used as forms of associative memory. The patterns of images stored in them correspond to stable states of nonlinear systems and to the local minima of functions representing the "energy" of the network. The memory capacity or the permitted number of image samples stored depends on the network size. The most popular recurrent networks are the Hopfield net and a BAM (bidirectional associative memory) network.
2. Multilayer feedforward neural networks. Information flows through such networks in one direction. These networks perform a non-linear mapping of input signals and output signals (which most frequently have the form of multidimensional vectors both on the input and the output). The most popular feedforward networks are the multi-layer perceptron trained using methods with

back error propagation (to more effectively train neurons of hidden layers) and the RBF (Radial Basis Functions) network which uses radial neurons (with a non-monotonous transition function) in the hidden layer.

3. SOM – self organizing maps. These networks operate by the rule of competitive learning. Output neurons compete one with another to get activated. The input signal is fed only to the winning neuron. Examples of such networks and Kohonen and ART networks.

Regardless of the great variety of neural networks, all of them include the components listed below in their structure.

- A finite number of neurons $x(1), x(2), \dots x(n)$, of which every one has its individual way of operating within the time t defined by its output signal $x_t(i)$.
- A finite number of connections between neurons $W=(w_{ij})$, where w_{ij} determines the weight of the connection between neuron $x(i)$ and neuron $x(j)$.
- A function for aggregating the input signal $\tau_t(i) = \sum_{j=1}^{n} x_t(j) w_{ij}$
- The activation function f for which τ is the input value generating as the output another output signal (or state) of the neuron $x_{t+1}(i) = f(\tau_t(i) - \theta)$, where θ is called the threshold and f is a nonlinear function, for example of the sigmoid type.

Networks most widely used for problems of identifying and classifying medical images are Kohonen and Hopfield networks as well as multi-layer perceptrons.

6.6.1. Kohonen network

The Kohonen network, also called a self-organizing feature map, is the most popular type of a self-organizing network.

A Kohonen network exhibits competitive learning, and the network itself is usually feedforward. Neurons are connected to all the components of an N-dimensional input vector X. The weights of neural connections make up the vector $wi = (w_{i1}, w_{i2}, \dots w_{in})T$. Before the learning process can start, the input signal vector X is normalized $||X||=1$, which can also be written as:

$$x_1 = \frac{x_1}{\sqrt{\sum_{v=1}^{n} (x_v)^2}}$$

When the network is stimulated by vector X, a competition starts and is won by the neuron whose weights are the least different from the appropriate components of the stimulating vector. The winning neuron, therefore, fulfils the relationship $d(x, w_w) = \min_{1<i<n} d(x, w_i)$

The distance between vector x and vector w is represented as $d(x, w)$. A topological neighborhood of the winning neuron $Sw(n)$ is also adopted, and its radius shrinks over time. Then an adaptation process occurs between the winning neuron and the neighboring ones in accordance with the Kohonen rule:

$$w_i(n+1) = w_i(n) + \eta_i(n)[x - w_i(n)]$$

$\eta_i(n)$ is the coefficient of the ith neuron from the neighborhood $Sw(n)$, whose value decreases along with the distance from the winning neuron, while the weights of neurons from outside the neighborhood stay the same.

Kohonen's learning algorithm has the following form:

$$w_i(n+1) = w_i(n) + \eta G(i,x)[x - w_i(n)]$$

The learning coefficient of every neuron i is separated from its distance from vector x included in $G(i,x)$ which represents the neighborhood function. Function $G(i,x)$ is defined as follows:

$$G(i,x)\begin{cases} 1 \text{ when } & d(i,w) \le \lambda \\ 0 \text{ else} \end{cases}$$

$d(i,w)$ is the Euclidean distance from the winning neuron w to the ith neuron. Coefficient λ is the radius of the neighborhood, whose value decreases over time.

Such a neighborhood is referred to as rectangular. The second type of a neighborhood found in Kohonen networks is the Gaussian neighborhood for which:

$$G(i,x) = \exp\left(-\frac{d^2(i,w)}{2\lambda^2}\right)$$

The Euclidean distance and the radius of the neighborhood determine the adaptation degree of neurons from the neighborhood of the winning one. In practice, the Gaussian network is preferable, as it yields better learning results and a better network organization [54].

6.6.2. Hopfield net

A Hopfield net is a recurrent net forming a type of an associative memory. It is usually presented as a system with an output feedback, meaning that output signals of neurons are at the same time input signals of the network. In the classical layout of a Hopfield net we omit the feedback to the neuron from its own output, so the matrix of weights is as symmetric as shown in Figure 6.9.

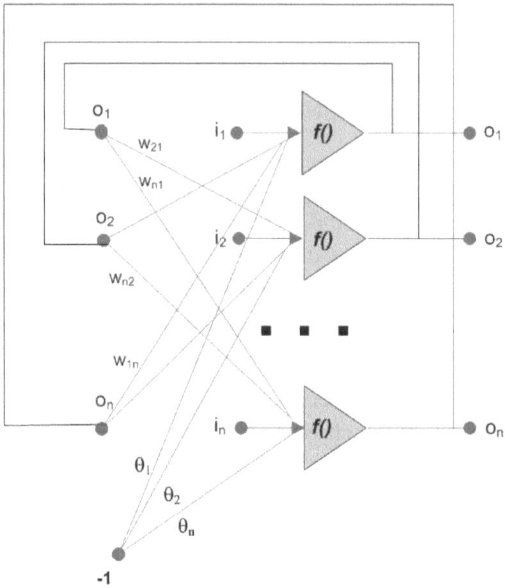

Fig. 6.9. A Hopfield net diagram

For a network to act as an associative memory, it has to be trained in a special way. For that purpose weights W_{ij} of particular neurons must be selected so that during the recovery, the network is able to find the dataset closest to the testing vector. This process causes an area of attraction to be created between particular balance points which correspond to the training data. In the case of a network with an associative memory, we are dealing with a single vector or a set of such which, by training, determines the location of particular attractors. It is assumed that every neuron has an activation function of the signum type which takes the value of ± 1, and as a result the output signal of the ith neuron can be described by the function below:

$$y_i = \operatorname{sgn}\left(\sum_{j=0}^{N} w_{ij} x_j + b_i \right)$$

It should also be assumed that the constant component of polarization which defines the operation of particular networks is a component of the input vector x. If we omit the unit delays of the network which represent the synchronic mode of signal transmitting, dependencies describing the network can be presented in the following form (for the initial condition $y(0) = x$)

$$y_i(k) = \operatorname{sgn}\left(\sum_{j=1, i \neq j}^{N} w_{ij} y_j(k-1) \right)$$

Two modes of operation of a Hopfield net can be distinguished: the learning mode and the recovery mode. In the learning mode, weights w_{ij} are selected based on the set training patterns x. In the recovery mode, assuming the initial state of the neuron $y(0) = x$ and at set values of weights, a transitory process occurs which ends in the defined local minimum where $y(n) = y(n-1)$. During the presentation of a single training pattern x, changes will continue until the above relationship is fulfilled for all neurons.

The associative memory provided by a Hopfield net has corrective features. If the test sample presented differs by a certain number of bits, the network can correct these bits and complete the classification process in the appropriate attractor. An associative memory has its specific capacity which is understood as the maximum number of patterns stored and recovered with the minimum error of e_{max}.

It has been shown that using the Hebb rule for training and allowing a relative error of $e_{max} = 1\%$, the maximum capacity of the memory represents just 13.8% of neurons forming the associative memory.

6.6.3. Multi-layer perceptron

Perceptrons are networks built of layers of regularly interconnected neurons. Every input of a neuron from one layer is connected to the outputs of all neurons from the previous layer (Figure 6.10).

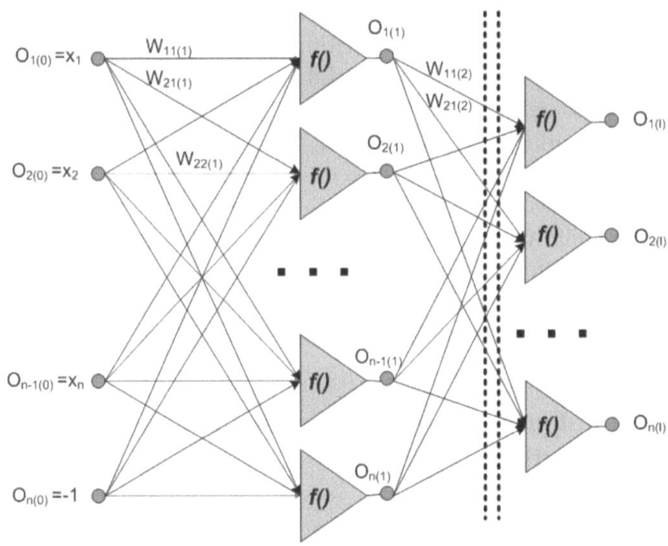

Fig. 6.10. The diagram of a multi-layer network

The number of neurons in a layer and the number of layers are unrestricted. In a special case, the perceptron can be built of a single layer and a single neuron, although perceptrons applied to practical image classification problems are multilayer. Their first layer is called the input layer and the last one the output layer, while the remaining layers are called hidden. The number of hidden layers is unrestricted, but in practice it is usually no greater than two so as to keep the computing time short.

The method of training with back error propagation is used to train a network containing at least one hidden layer. This method is among the most popular for training multi-layer networks and has contributed to a significant extension of the range of applications of artificial neural networks. The model with back error propagation consists of three neural layers. The input and output layers contain the same number of neurons, while the hidden layer usually contains fewer. There is no feedback in the structure of this model, and the activation function is of a sigmoid type.

$$f(NET) = \frac{1}{1+\exp(-NET)}$$

Training using the back error propagation method can be applied for a network with any number of layers, of which at least two must have the values of weights set in them.

The purpose is to set the values of weights in such a way that after stimulating with a certain set of input vectors we can get the desired set of output vectors. Training pairs, each of which contains an input vector and its corresponding output vector, called the target vector, are used. The set of all pairs constitutes the training set. Before the training process can start, all weights must be initiated as low random values to prevent neurons entering the saturation state at a later stage.

The training process itself runs in the following way: the next pair is selected from the training set and the stimulating vector is fed to the network input. Then, the state at the network output is calculated. Then the error between the value of the target vector and the value calculated on the output of the network is defined and the values of network weights are set one after another so that the error is minimized. The entire operations runs until the error for the entire set is small enough. Calculations are made layer after layer, starting with the input layer. After the identification has been completed, the output state which represents the result looked for is determined on the outputs of neurons of the output layer.

6.7. Bayesian and other probabilistic methods of pattern recognition in medical applications

Traditional image recognition methods can also include probabilistic methods. Just as in the case of neural networks, recognition algorithms can be divided into supervised and unsupervised methods. Supervised recognition takes place when the recognition applies to pre-set patterns. This type of recognition can be subdivided into smaller groups of methods, such as:

- The maximum probability method
- The Bayes method
- The minimum distance classifier (described above)

- The entropy criterion

Unsupervised recognition occurs when it is done without reference to set patterns, which are not available in this case. This group of methods can be split into subgroups which include:

- Isodata, k-means or c-means grouping;
- Vector quantizing;
- Hierarchical clustering.

Statistical classification algorithms assign patterns to the most probable classes. The rules of decision making can be formulated in many ways. We usually take into account the value of the classification error and the transformation of the probability $P(w_i)$ – known by assumption and related to the class – into the probability $P(w_i|x)$, where x is the n-dimensional vector.

Recognizing images with statistical methods is based on the assumption that for every class, the probabilities $P(w_i|x)$ and $P(w_i)$ are known. In addition, the class number must be known by assumption. We also have a set of training samples which represent the type of features and the principal classes, where every one of them has the same label as the class corresponding to it.

This is where the training problem arises. If the form of density is known, we have the problem of defining the parameter. Bayes method represents one of the ways to determine probability density functions based on the available experimental data described by the feature vector corresponding to the patterns of the training samples. Every probability density function (PDF) may be characterised by the appropriate set of parameters.

The most broadly used is the Gauss function characterized by mean values and the covariance matrix which is defined for every class w_i contained in the training data set. This technique is called parametric estimation.

Examples of parametric estimation comprise two methods: the maximum probability method and the Bayes method.

The maximum probability method assumes that parameters are constant, but are not known. It finds the best parameters which increase the probability of obtaining a given training set.

The Bayes method uses the training set to update the training set dependent on the density function of unknown parameters. The training set allows a priori information to be replaced with empirically determined density functions.

6.7.1. Bayes method

Bayesian decision-making theory constitutes the basic statistical method used to classify images. The technique is based on the assumption that the problem for decision-making is formulated in a probabilistic way and significant probabilistic parameters are set.

The best way of illustrating this issue is to present it with reference to the example of two classes *w1,w2*. The a priori probabilities of these classes $P(w_1)$ and $P(w_2)$ are known by assumption from the moment when they can be distinguished from the available training set. Probability density distribution functions $p(x_i|w_i)$, $i=1, 2$ are also known.

$p(x_i|w_i)$ can also be called the function of the conditional probability of *w1* with reference to x_i .

By referring to the Bayes principle we get $P(w_i \mid x) = \dfrac{p(x \mid w_i)P(w_i)}{p(x)}$

where $p(x)$ is the distribution of the probability x, to which the following formula applies:

$$p(x) = \sum_{i=1}^{2} p(x \mid w_i)P(w_i)$$

Bayes classification principle is easiest to discuss for two classes w_1 w_2. The following rules apply then:

If $P(w1|x) > P(w2|x)$, then x is determined for *w1*

If $P(w1|x) < P(w2|x)$, then x is determined for *w2*

Figure 6.11 shows two equally probable classes and their probability density functions $p(x|w_i)$. The vertical line marks the threshold dividing a single-dimensional feature space into two regions R1 and R2. According to Bayes rule, all values of x belonging to R1 are determined for class *w1*, and values x belonging to R2 are determined for class *w2*.

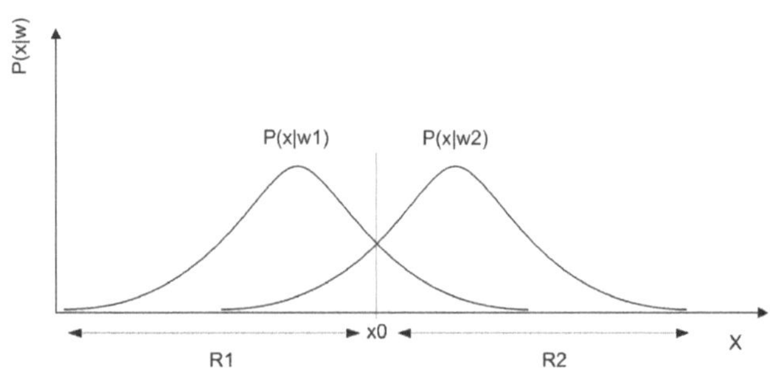

Fig. 6.11. A diagram of classification with the Bayes rule

The probability of committing a decision-making error can be determined from the following formula:

$$Pe = \int_{-\infty}^{x_0} p(x \mid w_2)dx + \int_{x_0}^{+\infty} p(x \mid w_1)dx$$

The classification error is at the minimum when features are divided into two regions R1 and R2 in the following way:

R1: P(w1|x) > P(w2|x)
R2: P(w2|x) > P(w1|x)

Obviously, the reasoning presented above for two classes can be generalized for M classes $w_1, w_2, w_3, \ldots w_m$. Then, the feature vector x is assigned to class w_i when:

$$P(w_i \mid x) > P(w_j \mid x) \;\; \forall j \neq i$$

Every time an object is assigned to a class, there is a risk of making a wrong identification. Wrong identifications can be defined using the alleged cost function. Let $L(i, j)$ be the cost (loss) resulting from the wrong assignment of an object to class i, when that object belongs to class j. Under such assumptions, the wrong classification can be assessed by defining the alleged cost function $L(i, j)$ where i, j = 1,2,...M. This function $L(i, j)$ is equal to zero if the feature vector x is assigned to the right class and is greater than zero in the other case, i.e. $L(i,j) > 0$ when x is assigned to class w_j instead of the right class w_i. When considering wrong classifications in terms of the losses incurred, the conditional loss parameter $Ri(x)$ with regard to assigning x to a class can be defined as:

$$R_i(x) = \sum_{j=1}^{M} L(i, j) P(w_j \mid x)$$

or synonymously

$$R_i(x) = \sum_{j=1}^{M} L(i, j) p(x \mid w_j) P(w_j)$$

For practical applications, the following assumptions are made: $L(i, j) = 0$ if $i = j$ and $L(i,j) = 1$ if $i \neq j$.

On the basis of the above conclusions and definitions, we get a slightly changed principle of Bayes classification which states that the feature vector x is assigned to class w_i for which $Ri(x)$ is at the minimum.

6.7.2. An example of using Bayes classification to recognize tumors

When recognizing cancerous lesions, we consider only two states: the normal state and the state with cancerous lesions present.

We therefore need to consider two differentiating functions: $f_{abnormal}(x)$ and $f_{normal}(x)$. The classified case is assigned to the abnormal state if $f_{abnormal}(x) > f_{normal}(x)$. Assuming that the a priori probabilities are equal for every class, based on formula [26]

$$f_i(x) = -\frac{1}{2}(x - \mu_i)^T \Sigma_i^{-1} (x - \mu_i') + \ln P(w_i) + c_i$$

we get the following function differentiating states for recognizing tumors:

$$f(x) = -\frac{1}{2}(x-\mu)^T \Sigma^{-1}(x-\mu) + \log|\Sigma|$$

If each of these states has a distribution which uses the same covariance matrix, the decision areas of *abnormal* and *normal* may be separated one from the other with a hyperplane in the space *x*. Consequently, the classifier resulting from the Bayes criterion is frequently presented as a linear classifier. However, if the covariance matrixes are not equal, then the decision-making plane is formed of hypersquare surfaces, and the classifier is presented as a hypersquare classifier.

6.7.3. Maximum entropy criterion

The definition of entropy comes from the Shannon information theory and in image recognition applications means the measure of the randomness of feature vectors. Entropy *H* for the probability density function *p(x)* is defined by the following formula:

$$H = -\int_X p(x)\ln p(x)dx$$

In addition, it is necessary to assume that *p(x)* is unknown but some boundary data (means, variances) is known.

To better understand this, it is worth presenting it using an example.

Let us assume that the random variable x is different from zero for $a \le x \le b$ and is equal to zero outside this interval. We want to determine the maximum entropy of its probability density function. In this sense, it is necessary to determine the maximum of the above formula of entropy assuming that:

$$\int_a^b p(x)dx = 1$$

Using Lagrange multipliers, we obtain the synonymous form [26]

$$H_L = -\int_a^b p(x)(\ln p(x) - \lambda)dx$$

Derivative H_L related to *p(x)* is defined by the formula

$$\frac{\partial H_L}{\partial p(x)} = -\int_a^b \{(\ln p(x) - \lambda) + 1\}dx$$

Equating the above formula to zero gives us

$$\hat{p}(x) = \exp(\lambda - 1)$$

The assumptions indicate that $\exp(\lambda - 1) = \frac{1}{b-a}$. The value of the probability *p(x)* we are looking for, for which the entropy reaches its maximum, can therefore be determined from the formula

$$p(x) = \begin{cases} \dfrac{1}{b-a} & a \le x \le b \\ 0 & else \end{cases}$$

It is easy to see that the requirement to achieve the maximum entropy of an unknown distribution of probability *p(x)* is satisfied when *p(x)* is a uniform (rectangular) distribution on a certain interval.

6.7.4. Non-parametric estimation methods

In contrast to parametric estimation methods, in non-parametric estimation we do not have much data that we can use directly. In the majority of problems of image recognition we have no information on probability density functions related to the classes, so they have to be estimated directly on the basis of the data. There are many methods based on non-parametric estimation. Some of them rely on estimating the density function $p(x|w_i)$ based on trial patterns. If results achieved this way turn out to be good, they can be integrated with the optimum classifier. Another way is to estimate directly on the basis of a posteriori probabilities $P(w_i|x)$. This method more related to non-parametric decision-making procedures which omit probability estimation and perform decision-making functions directly.

The following methods are the most useful and popular:

- The histogram method
- Parzen Windows
- *k*-Nearest Neighbor
- The potential function method

6.7.5. Histogram method

This is the simplest and most popular method for estimating the probability density function. To apply it, we generally need no theoretical premises, but to obtain reliable results, we need a relatively large sample with a data set allowing us to build the necessary statistics. Let us see how that works.

For a simple, one-dimensional case, the *x* axis is split into intervals *h* long, and for every interval, the probability of a sample *x* contained in it is determined.

Let *N* be the total number of samples, and k_N the number of samples belonging to a certain interval. The probability of the appropriate classes is then defined by the formula $P \approx k_N / N$.

This method of proceeding is illustrated in Figure 6.12.

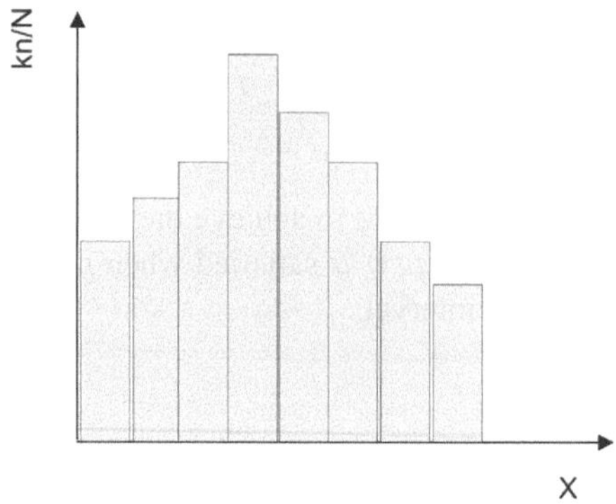

Fig. 6.12. The histogram method

The generalization of this method of proceeding to a multidimensional case is notionally simple, but due to the quick rise of the number of intervals which require their k_N values to be determined for multidimensional spaces, this method is of a rather marginal practical utility.

6.7.6. Parzen windows

This is the most important of all non-parametric methods. For its better understanding let us again consider a simple, one-dimensional case. The purpose will be to estimate the value of the function of density *p(x)* at point *x*.

This requires determining the number of samples N_h falling within the interval around point *x* *[x – h, x + h]*. Such values have to be established for every point *x* and then divided by the total number of feature vectors *M* and the length of the interval, i.e. the value of *2h*. The above procedure yields an estimated value of the density function looked for at point *x*.

$$p(x) = \frac{N_h(x)}{2hM}$$

As the supporting function K_h we select:

$$K_h = \begin{cases} 0,5 & |m| \leq 1 \\ 0 & |m| > 1 \end{cases}$$

The substitution produces

$$p(x) = \frac{1}{hM} \sum_{i=1}^{M} K\left(\frac{x - m_i}{h} \right)$$

together with the ith component of the sum equal to zero if m_i exceeds the interval *[x – h, x + h]*.

Finally, it leads us to the following form of the relationshi p: $\gamma(x,m) = \frac{1}{h}K\left(\frac{x-m}{h}\right)$. These values have been presented in Figure 6.13.

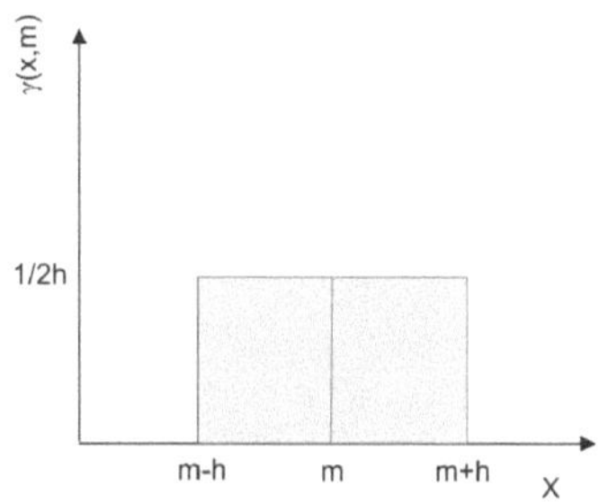

Fig. 6.13. Grouping a table of two-dimensional vectors. The maximum number of vectors in one group is 7 [26]

If $p(x)$ is considered as a function consistent with the number of samples, we get $p(x) = p(x,M)$

Parzen has proven that the estimation of the value of p for $M \rightarrow \infty$ is free of deviations if $h = h(M)$ and $\lim\limits_{M \longrightarrow \infty} h(M) = 0$.

In practice, when we only have a finite number of samples, we have to choose the right values of M and h. It is good to start with a preliminary estimation of h, and then change it to minimize the likelihood of an error occurring in the assignment. Theoretically, we need a large M to get a greater effectiveness of identification, but in practice a large number of data points needlessly increases the computational complexity of the classifier.

6.7.7. Application of probabilistic methods

Recognition based on the statistical techniques described in this chapter is mainly used in oncology, particularly to detect breast tumors in mammography examinations (Fig. 6.14).

In such examinations, every case is identified based on four images, showing both breasts of the patient in two views. One view is taken from top down, the other from the side. Getting two independent projections provides a better visualization of the potentially threatened regions, which may be shown differently in independent images. In his/her analyzes, the diagnostician looks for characteristic lesions indicating the presence of a tumor. Among those lesions, the presence of grouped microcalcifications can be distinguished. In general, statistical methods are considered to be of poor precision, although this obviously depends on the specific case, but they are not used too widely and are usually treated as a kind of verification indicator for the hypotheses made. They are therefore often helpful to verify the correctness of results achieved using methods other than statistical algorithms.

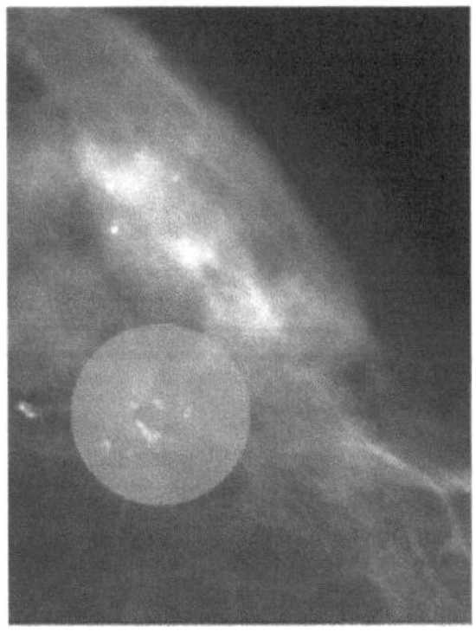

Fig. 6.14. Examples of images from mammography examinations showing microcalcifications

6.8. Syntactic and other structural methods in medical image recognition

The mathematical methods presented in the previous chapters of this book, regardless of their complexity and sophistication, are not very efficient in some cases. This is particularly obvious when we analyze images that are very complex and for which the number of classes is very large (this leads to a great increase in the dimension of feature spaces used to describe the patterns). However, syntactic methods of image recognitions which use the formalisms of mathematical linguistics are free of such limitations [55].

In the syntactic approach, the complex image is divided into simpler sub-images, and then an attempt is made to recognize them using holistic methods, treating those sub-images as independent units. If the sub-images are highly complex, the splitting operation is continued until we get the picture primitives. Picture primitives are indivisible elements of the image which we assume to exist and be capable of defining for a given image class.

So in the case of syntactic methods, before we undertake the recognition as such, we have to distinguish the picture primitives as well as the relationships between them. The most widespread method of distinguishing picture primitives is to segment the image using such methods as: edge detection using gradient operators or pattern matching operators. The identification of patterns is an immensely important stage, since when recognizing images (or picture primitives in this case), we treat them as independent images. Consequently, the correct assembly of sub-images into the whole image is the condition for its correct recognition (Fig. 6.15).

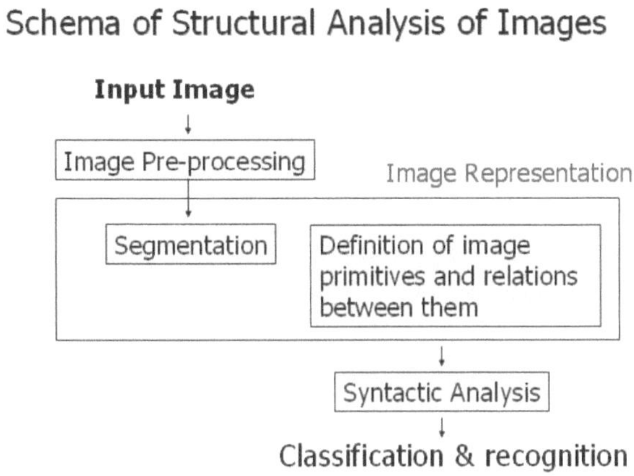

Fig. 6.15. A diagram of structural image recognition

Apart from picture primitives, another important step of the recognition procedure in the syntactic approach to recognizing a picture is to determine the relationships between picture primitives. This is because those relationships are the conditions for the correct assembly of the image, and therefore for its correct recognition. The nature of the relationship also represents a very important criterion of the basic classification of syntactic methods of image recognition.

Syntactic image recognition methods are classified into three main formal methods. The first and earliest to be developed are *sequence methods*. The more sophisticated methods described further down are *tree methods* and *graph methods*.

The first group of methods to be developed are sequence methods in which the image is represented by a sequence, so we distinguish one type of relationship which may occur between picture primitives. This relationship is concatenation of another element. Sequence languages are designed for recognizing and describing single (sometimes very complicated) image objects. Examples of such languages are: languages based on chain codes (Freeman's), image description languages (Shaw's) and languages describing shape features (Jakubowski's) [54]. However, the above languages are incapable of describing multi-object images. This capability is offered by tree and graph languages. Sequence formalisms have been successfully used to analyze medical images. Special cases of recognizing various complicated shapes of organs in the abdominal cavity and the chest are presented in [55]. Types of such applications are also presented in Figure 6.16.

Tree methods are built on the basis of tree languages.Two types of applications of those methods are the most popular: scene analysis and texture analysis. Scene analysis is a process of recognizing a 3D image in which objects constituting its components have been distinguished and identified, and relationships between such objects have been described. We distinguish two sets of picture primitives.

The first set describes the objects making up the image, the second describes the relationships that may occur between objects (Fig. 6.17).

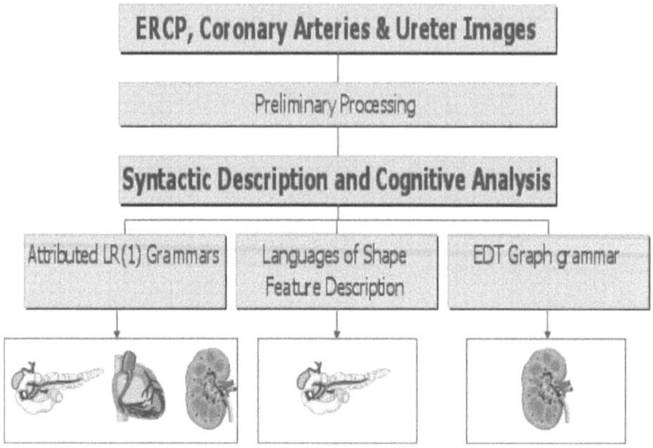

Fig. 6.16. Examples of images and medical structures recognized with structural image analysis methods [55]

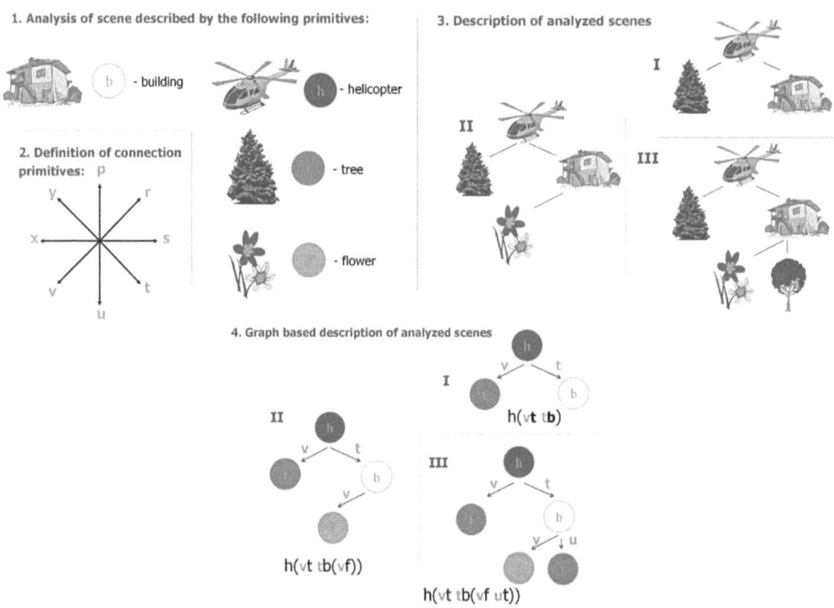

Fig. 6.17. A graph description of the analyzed image containing several objects. 1) Objects recognized independently, 2) relationships between particular elements of the scene, 3) examples of similar scenes, 4) tree descriptions of the images recognized

Graph grammars represent the most robust tools used to recognize images. This is why the use of graphs to describe 2D or 3D images is commonly found in the literature. However, their application for recognizing medical images is not that widespread, as the syntactic analysis of graph grammars, and more precisely, the computational complexity of the syntactic analysis problem poses a lot of difficulty. However, further chapters of this book will present examples of using such methods, which concern analyzing palm images and spatial reconstructions of coronary vessels.

7. Automatic understanding of medical images as a new paradigm for advanced computer aiding of medical investigations

Medical procedures based on this or that use of various images have become a subject of great importance and interest for computer science. This is because contemporary medical diagnostics is increasingly based on various forms of imaging. Today, technologies collectively labeled as Medical Imaging represent a leading source of information used both in contemporary treatment techniques and research, whether in medicine, biology or biomedical engineering. This information may concern both the morphology of the organs analyzed and their function, as some types of medical imaging support the presentation of an image of functional (and not just morphological) properties of a given organ: PET or fMRI. Images combining good morphological imaging (e.g. CT) with a modern topographic functional examination (e.g. PET) are increasingly used allows one to formulate conclusions on the correct or pathological course of biological processes running within the observed structures. Nowadays, such a combined set of image information increasingly frequently forms the foundation for the scientific reasoning or the process of diagnostic reasoning in the present meaning of the term.

Earlier chapters of this book have shown how medical images can be acquired, processed, analyzed and recognized. Further down in this chapter, we will present a new, original approach which the authors of this book have been proposing for several years, leading to the automatic **understanding of medical images**, in a way similar to how a physician can understand these images and, based on them, draw conclusions about the nature of the observed disease process and the way in which this pathology can be overcome using various therapeutic methods.

As a research concept, automatic image understanding is still new and not accepted by some researchers. It builds on advanced techniques of computational intelligence. In this concept, we use cognitive reasoning mechanisms which are a world apart from all image recognition techniques described in the previous chapter. These techniques are clearly novel compared to all the known, classical methods of image classification, as they make it possible to achieve automatic machine perception of a much deeper nature than in all the previous techniques. In typical recognition techniques, you first build an arbitrary list of classes (categories) to which the object considered may belong and then you conduct the whole image analysis in such a way as to determine in which of these classes the object can be included. In contrast to this very formal procedure, in the automatic understanding of medical images we try to reach the semantic meaning of all details detected as a result of analyzing the image. One result of this insight into the subdestantive content of the image and the attempt to understand the nature of processes which have led to the that particular appearance of the organ in question in this image, could be the determination of the disease entity to which the analyzed medical problem should be classified. This would make automatic understanding a

M.R. Ogiela and R. Tadeusiewicz: *Automatic understanding of medical images as a new paradigm for advanced computer aiding of medical investigations,* Studies in Computational Intelligence (SCI) **84**, 153–170 (2007)
www.springerlink.com

very valuable tool aiding the diagnostic process. However, understanding the nature of a disease entails richer content than the simple automatic classification which mechanically assigns the disease name to the patient, so we claim that automatic medical image understanding offers a significantly novel meaning and presents new opportunities in a field in which automatic recognition was until recently considered the limit of computer deployment. We will try to further develop and substantiate this thesis in the sections below.

7.1. A general overview of the image understanding concept

Nature has equipped us with the ability to understand. We understand what is said to us, we understand written text, we understand the situation we are in, we understand (or rather attempt to) other people. In everyday intellectual activities, we do not ponder what the word "understanding" really means, just use our understanding of something or focus our effort to get to understand it.

The need for a new look at the problems of understanding appeared as information technology tried to gatecrash this discipline. Many a time has our wish to entrust more and more fields of our own information activities to computers put us in a position in which an operation apparently obvious and generally understood, performed by men frequently and without giving much thought to its nature, suddenly became really mysterious and escaped the precise definition when we faced the need to delegate it to machines. It is worth noting that typical information operations, such as making calculations, processing text, collecting data, communicating and transferring information never led to such discussions or provoked such problems. It seems that one of the reasons for this easy acceptance and assimilation of the achievements of traditional information technology was that even in the pre-IT era, i.e. when people had no access to computers, they used various props from the outside world: an abacus, a printing press, a library file or the telegraph. So a computer database may be huge, very useful and even very costly, but it is by no means mystical: it is only a filing system, just very big and easy to use.

However, when we try to apply information technology to activities for which the natural toolbox is inside our mind and is represented by the rather mysterious screen of our consciousness, emotions explode and in order to keep the resulting debates and disputes in order, we need very precise definitions, as without them, many of the discussions get bogged down on various planes, in the very negative meaning of the word. This negative multi-planar nature is due to every disputant putting the problem on his/her own plane, which does not intersect the planes of other disputants, and defends his/her views with arguments that are true only in his/her own plane. Let us remember the violent debates about the existence artificial intelligence as such or the lack thereof, let's quote the somewhat old hat debate as to whether a machine can think, let's note how deep an analysis and reform was needed for the activity of image recognition when it turned out that, for many reasons, we needed to automate it.

It seems that now we are ready for another iteration of this dispute. On the surface, this is a purely academic dispute referring to the semiotics and the theory of meanings, but in fact, it is a dispute about the limits of automating intellectual processes, and its resolution will have both theoretical value and major practical importance.

The subject to be debated is the capacity (as the enthusiasts would call it) or the impossibility (as conservatives would) of **automatic understanding.**

No one needs convincing that understanding brings measurable benefits. That typical computer applications, even the fanciest ones, are by no means capable of really understanding those huge resources and streams of information that computers capture, store, send and process is something we know from our everyday frustrations with the computers we use.

This is why more and more is now being said about the need to develop, as a new field in artificial intelligence, a technique for the automatic understanding of various bits of information swarming somewhere out there behind the computer screen. This need was first discovered by specialists analyzing textual information. The subjects of semantic networks, information searches based on various onthologies, automatic translation of documents written in one language into another, and the automatic generation of summaries of lengthy texts inescapably led to reaching deeper than just the lexical layer of the texts in question. Having sorted out (to a better of worse extent) the syntactic problems stemming from the complicated structure of natural language grammars, it became necessary to face up to the semantic aspect, which is the barrier between the two spheres: of the **meanings** of specific pieces of information, many times richer and more difficult, and of their **signs**, so nice and easy to automatically process using computers

But that is not all. Some 10 years ago, the authors, supported by a group of co-workers (but also with the active contribution from their competitors) introduced the concept of **automatic image understanding** into the global literature.

Contrary to appearances, the images viewed have not only their **form** but also their **content.**

The form can be improved using computers and digital image processing applications, until recently available only to huge labs which refined images from space probes or various espionage devices, but now also to a layman refining snapshots from Aunt Helen's birthday party. **The form** of an image can also be analyzed by automatically calculating various parameters of objects visible in it, and classified, for example using the functionalities provided by neuron networks generally available these days.

However, so far we have no tools for penetrating the content of an image. The visual part of our brain can process signals from vision receptors very efficiently as it can very rapidly *generalize* the video information to a contextual cognitive map of the recognized objects and the relationships between them. This form of scene description is referred to as *high-level*, in contrast to the *low-level* representation made up of the set of impressions recorded by the retina. The brain does not create subsequent versions of photographs of the world around us, but knowledge-based models with a preference for the meaning of the situation observed and not its form (which is of secondary importance). In computer systems, we also need to try to extract the substantive meaning of the acquired image instead of running one algorithm after another to transform sequences of values of particular points (*pixels*) of the image obtained by its direct acquisition in increasingly sophisticated ways.

Further down in this chapter we will discuss the fundamental concept of **automatic understanding,** at first from a more general perspective, to organize and compile the relevant notions. The title and contents of the whole book indicate that we will mainly propose tools for the automatic understanding of the semantic content of **medical images.** Regardless of such a limitation of our analysis, the methods developed will be presented in a way allowing us to obtain better quality ways of using image information in a broad range of various applications of techniques collectively referred to as *computer vision.* We can hope that, by giving a **specific** example of how to overcome the barrier between the form and the content of images, we will encourage more researchers to look for ways to overcome that barrier for other signals: for example geophysical signals in prospecting for underground deposits of valuable resources or mechanical signals to detect the first symptoms of impending failures of crucial equipment, e.g. an airplane engine.

Let us, however, return to medical images. The progress in medical imaging technologies and ceaseless efforts of engineers trying to find more and more ways of acquiring and presenting information on the shapes and functions of human internal organs have given us the present huge number of various medical image types. Today's biomedical engineering not only provides the physician with all these images of internal organs and the processes running in them, but uses advanced information technology, collectively referred to as *computer vision*, to refine, assess and classify these images. These subject have been discussed above in this book, so they need no detailed discussing here, but to put the proposed methods of automatic image understanding in the right context, we should note that *computer vision,* at its current development stage, offer three types of computer image handling methods:

- *Image processing* – aimed at image **quality improvement** and distinguishing only **objects** of medical interest from the whole complex image (e.g. by segmentation);
- *Image analysis* – aimed at defining the features of the entire image or particular objects distinguished in it as well as counting objects and calculating the **values** of their quantitative features or assigning **category names** to their quantitative features;
- *Pattern recognition* – aimed at identifying and classifying elements or regions distinguished within images by indexing them as objects belonging to some pre-selected classes, mainly on the basis of their shape, size or characteristics of their shading (texture).

The relationships and dependencies between medical image handling techniques and the techniques of image semantics understanding, discussed further down, are presented in Figure 7.1.

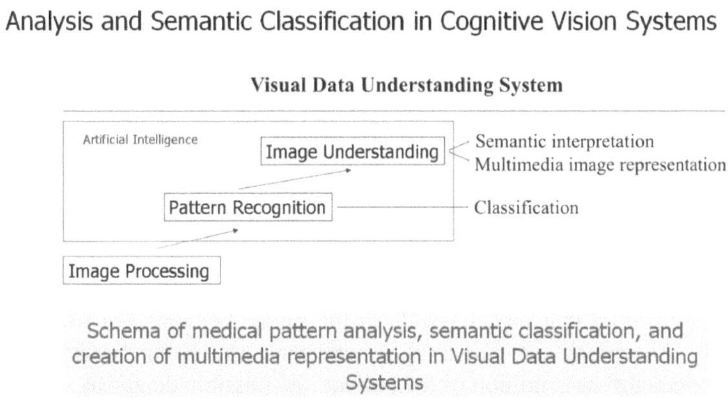

Fig. 7.1. Interrelationships between classical elements of the image interpretation process and image understanding techniques defined further below

Traditional recognition methods have been presented in earlier chapters of this book. It is only worth noting that all three stages of the "traditional" computer processing of medical images are used more and more frequently, which makes them of key importance for the whole field of biomedical engineering. In particular, these techniques have become useful tools supporting and improving doctors' work, as image processing and refinement give physicians much better view of the details of examined organs and processes running in them, allowing them to make more apt diagnostic decisions with greater assurance. The results of all analyses of medical image characteristics and objects visible in them, generated by computers, allow the physician to base his/her reasoning on much more reliable and quantifiable premises than just a visual assessment of that image, improving both the effectiveness of his/her activities, and the feeling of reliability and security. Finally, the increasing acceptance of techniques for the automatic recognition and classification of biological objects distinguished in medical images can help the doctor make the right diagnostic decisions, although these techniques sometimes require the doctor to be able to critically assess the automatically suggested categories, as every recognition technique carries some level of error, while nothing excuses the doctor's personal responsibility for his/her decisions.

All those techniques for the computer processing, analysis and recognition of medical images do not, however, exhaust the full range of tasks and problems that may appear in connection with using an image as the source of useful diagnostic information. This is because in this entire field, it is data interpretation, which relates to the physician's knowledge, that is the most important and the most difficult job. At the present development stage of the technology discussed here, it is only the doctor's knowledge, including the knowledge of the regular and pathological anatomy and physiology of the analyzed organs and other parts of the body, that allows him or her to correctly understand the implications of this or that appearance of the medical image. Computer image processing may help make organ outlines and their changes caused by the disease process clearer and more precisely visible, but it is the doctor who must judge what follows from the fact that the image shows what it does.

The process of extracting and defining the characteristics of the image which accompany its automatic analysis and attempts at the automatic classification provides also just the premises for the reasoning process which the doctor has to conduct on the basis of his/her knowledge, imagination and frequently also intuition. Without this substantive interpretation of analytical results and automatic classification elements, they are in fact useless, as for the diagnostic and therapeutic procedure it makes no difference what value this or that image parameter has or to which class this or that object visible in the image belongs. For the doctor and, obviously, the patient, only one thing is important: what follows from all this with regard to the current condition of the patient, the possible diagnosis of the disease he/she is suffering from, the optimum plan of the therapy or rehabilitation and the projected results of its completion. All of the modern technology generating the numerous, varied medical images, as well as all the information technology included in classical *computer vision* methods is therefore dependent on one main factor, which is the process of medical **image interpretation** by a human.

Yet that process is getting more and more difficult for people as the numerous and complicated images provided by the technology require physicians to constantly gain new skills and qualifications for interpreting them, but usually the learning curve is less steep than that of the technological process. What is more, the progress in new medical imaging techniques usually replace the single image that the doctor used to view in the past to make the diagnosis with multiple images (a dozen or several dozen) for one patient, all of which have to be analyzed. For example, these numerous images present subsequent cross-sections of the brain tissue obtained by computed tomography or present the organ at different stages of absorbing or releasing the labeled pharmaceutical, or they show the same organ viewed with different imaging techniques etc. This obviously makes the diagnostic procedure much deeper and more detailed, but at the price of a huge increase in the effort of the physicians, who have to correctly interpret all these images, and to do so, they first have to correctly **understand** their contents.

In the light of the potential interpretation problems stemming from the constantly developed and therefore constantly changing modern medical visualization, the number of different organs that are examined and the many different ways in which disease processes can deform them, it is not surprising that image diagnostics urgently needs support from modern information technology. As a result, as the techniques for newer and newer forms of medical imaging develop, the demand grows for better and better techniques of computer assistance in the process of analyzing, interpreting, classifying and recognizing all these new images.

Nowadays, people increasingly expect that a modern medical system will not only acquire an image of the inside of a patient's body and will present it in the clearest possible way, but will also perform preliminary image analysis and will draw the physician's attention to only those elements which are most likely to carry information important for the diagnosis. This means that the computer not only has to compute (frequently in a very complex way) the values of each of the millions of pixels making up the image, but also has to intelligently analyze them and suggest to the doctor what they indicate. This is a challenge for IT specialists, who not only have to develop such new image analysis techniques, but also to constantly keep improving them.

This book is the product of several years of work by the authors, during which they developed and analyzed many methods of aiding the **substantive interpretation** of medical images. This aiding requires going "deep into" the substantive content of the analyzed medical images, which, in line with the concept presented in this book, boils down to two assumptions.

The first assumption is that **you can build a semantically-oriented (linguistic) description of the contents of a medical image** completely automatically, i.e. just on the basis of a properly conducted analysis of graphic structures detected in the image and their relationships. As a rule, this analysis has to follow a properly conducted procedure of preliminary image processing, which consists in running a sequence of routine image filtering, segmenting and transformations, selected so that image components significant for the interpretation are extracted, while technical disruptions and biological variability factors which make this semantically-oriented analysis difficult are limited or completely eliminated.

The second assumption says that a semantically-oriented description of image contents significant for a diagnosis can be confronted with properly expressed (in our case – contained in the structure of the appropriate graph grammar) **semantic expectations** and projections. The above semantic expectations result from our a-priori knowledge of the diagnostic or forecasting significance of specific structures shown in the analyzed class of medical images, so they are field-specific. This means that the right representation of the knowledge, which is the key to the automatic understanding of medical images, is not universal and has to be built separately for each class of medical problems. In other words, one has to have the appropriate representation of medical knowledge (e.g. the right graph grammar) created for every type of imaging, every organ and every type of disease. This is undoubtedly a lot of difficult work, but once it is completed, it can offer the function of **automatic understanding** of an increasingly broad class of medical images which will have a huge importance for the *medical imaging* technology, particularly in the hitherto neglected field of medical image interpretation, which extends the traditional triad of image processing, analysis and recognition.

This is important, as at the present stage of IT development we can easily process the **form** of the image using computers, but its **contents** remain almost completely impossible to automate. All processes for the practical application of vision information – also in medical systems – and the apparently simpler processes of searching for image information on a specific subject in large multimedia databases show the brutal truth that for images (unlike numbers or texts) **the form** of information can have very little connection to its **content.** It is particularly frequent that images **completely different in graphic terms** carry **the same content.** This is shown in Figure 7.2 which presents the same medical problem in the form of two completely different images recorded for two different patients, but leading to the very same diagnosis.

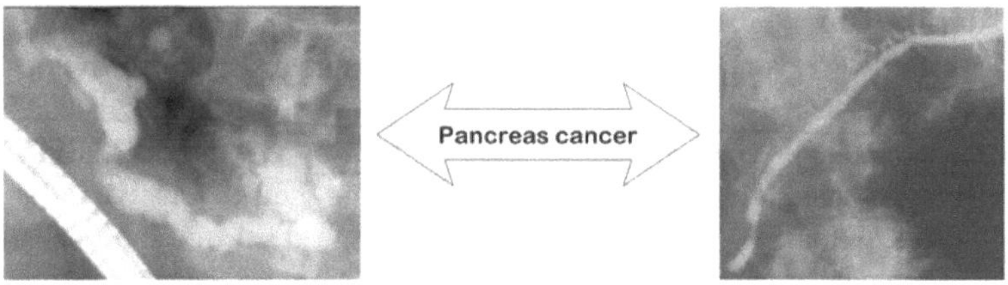

Fig. 7.2. Pancreatic cancer can be identified in both ERCP photographs, although these photographs are completely unlike each other

But if the form of the image is not identical to its content, we urgently need tools which would allow us to extract the semantic meaning of the image trapped in its complicated form. This automatic extraction of some important meaning which **is** present in the image, but in a trapped form is the purpose of **automatic image understanding** which the authors are proposing in this book and their other publications. The entrapment of the substantively important contents in the complicated (in the computer science sense) form of the image means that this content is not simply visible in the image, but its extraction and proper **understanding** requires some intellectual effort.

The difference between pattern recognition and image understanding includes the following assumptions:

- In recognition, we always have a fixed number of *a priori* known classes and all we need to do is to extract all these image features which are necessary and sufficient for the differentiation between the classes under consideration. After processing, we obtain the number (or name) of the proper class;
- In understanding, we do not have any *a priori* known classes or templates, because in fact the potential number of possible classes is infinite. So processing gives us a description of the image content based on no classification known *a priori*, as even the classification criteria are constructed and developed during the automatic reasoning process.

Now we will try to explain who and when can use this approach in the broad field of medical images.

7.2. Two-way data flow when solving image understanding problems

In this chapter we will try to explain what automatic image understanding is and how we can force the computer to understand image contents. Before we get down to details, we must demonstrate that there is in fact a fundamental difference between a formal description of an image (typically obtained by means of a variety of computer viewing methods) and the substantive meaning of the image, which can be discovered by an intelligent entity, capable of understanding the profound sense of the image in question.

To demonstrate such differences we need a method of extracting some kind of semantic content that is present in the image (picture), but that is not obviously noticeably in it. This task can be difficult as the gist is often hidden and needs a precise understanding of the image rather than its simple analysis, segmentation and even recognition. Based on the analyses of many unquestionably serious examples (medical images) we shall try to formulate the following three assumptions:

- The problem of the correct interpretation of many medical images cannot be solved by means of traditional image processing, image analysis or pattern recognition.
- The only way is to formulate a new paradigm of image interpretation and to develop a new method of its full automation, based on the application of advanced artificial intelligence tools.
- The automatic reasoning of image semantic contents, performed with the use of picture analysis, is referred to as automatic image understanding.

The fundamental features of automatic medical image understanding (which we postulate) can be listed as follows:

- We try to imitate the natural method in which a medical doctor thinks: he/she needs to understand the disease before making a formal diagnosis and choosing the right treatment.
- First we make a linguistic description of image contents, using a special kind of image description language. Using this idea, we can describe any image without specifying any limited number of *a priori* described classes.
- The linguistic description of the image content formulated in this manner forms the basis for a diagnosis based on understanding the image.

A very important difference between all traditional methods of automatic image processing (or recognition) and the new paradigm for image understanding is that in traditional methods data flows in only one direction, whereas there are two-way interactions between signals (features) extracted from image analysis and expectations resulting from the knowledge of image contents, as given by experts (physicians). Let us look at Fig. 7.3 which presents a traditional chart of image processing for medical purposes.

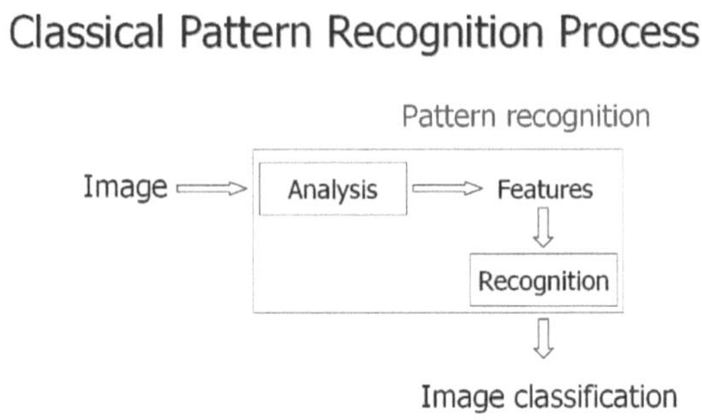

Fig. 7.3. Traditional method of medical image recognition

Unlike in this simple scheme representing the classical recognition, in the course of image understanding, information always flows both ways (Fig. 7.4).

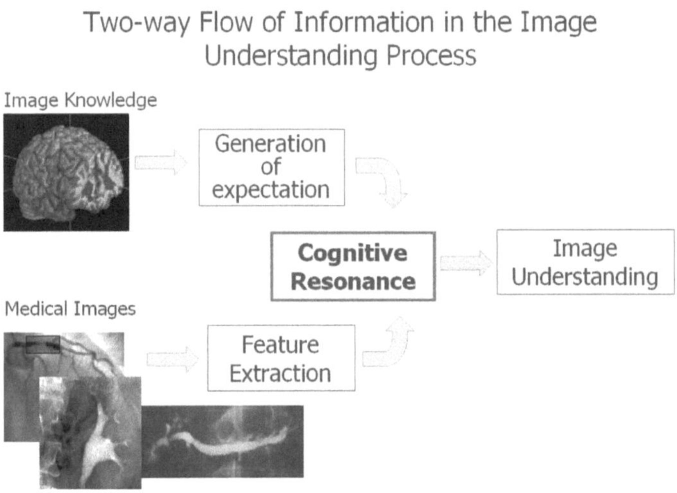

Fig. 7.4. The main paradigm of image understanding

Both above figures show that when we use the traditional pattern recognition paradigm, all processes of image analysis are based on a feed-forward scheme (a one-way flow of signals). In contrast, when we apply an automatic understanding of the image, the total input data stream (all features obtained by analysing the image under consideration) must be compared with the stream of **demands** generated by a dedicated **source of knowledge**. The demands are always connected with a specific (selected) hypothesis of the semantic interpretation of image contents. As a result, we can emphasise that the proposed 'demands' are a kind of postulates, describing (based on the knowledge about image contents) the desired values of some (selected) features of the image. The selected parameters of the image under consideration must have desired values when some assumption about semantic interpretation of the image content is to be validated as true. When the parameters of the input image are different – it **can** be interpreted as a **partial** falsification of one of the possible hypotheses about the meaning of the image content – but it still cannot be considered the final solution.

Due to this specific model of inference, we labelled our mechanism the 'cognitive resonance'. This name is appropriate to our ideas because during the comparison process of features calculated for the input image and demands generated by the source of knowledge, we can observe an amplification of some hypotheses (about the meaning of the image content) while other (competitive) hypotheses weaken. It is very similar to the interferential image formed during a mutual activity of two wave sources: at some points in space waves can add to one another, in other points there are of opposite phases and the final result is near zero.

Such a structure of the system for image understanding corresponds to one of very well known models of natural visual perception by man, named 'knowledge based perception'. The human eye cannot recognise an object if the brain has no template for such a likeness. This holds true even when the brain knows the object, but shown in another view, which means that other signals are coming to the visual cortex. Natural perception is, in fact, not just the processing of visual signals obtained by eyes. It is mainly a mental cognitive process, based on hypotheses generation and their real-time verification. The verification is performed by constantly comparing the selected features of an image with expectations derived from earlier visual experience.

Our method of image understanding is based on the same processes with the important difference that it is performed not by the physician but by computers.

7.3. Language description of the image as a key to understanding procedures

A very important aspect of the automatic image understanding method is the very close connection between our whole methodology and mathematical linguistics, especially a linguistic description of images. There are two important reasons for the selection of linguistic (syntactic) methods of image description as the fundamental tool for understanding images.

The first one is because (as has already been mentioned) in the case of understanding we have no limited number of classes or templates known *a priori*. In fact, when we try to understand an image we know nothing about, the possible number of potential classes reaches the infinity. So we must use a tool that offers functionalities to describe a potentially infinite number of categories. Moreover, the tool under consideration must be constructed from only a finite number of elements, as computers cannot operate using an infinite number of components. This means that it is necessary to have a tool which **generates** descriptions of classes rather than pointing to classes described *a priori*. For this reason, the only suitable tool is a language that can generate an infinite number of sentences on the basis of a finite number of components (words in vocabulary and rules in the grammar). Every other mechanism generating a finite list of identifiers or names will be absolutely insufficient in this case!

The second reason for using a linguistic approach to automatic image understanding is that this approach, after processing, yields a description of image contents making no use of any classification known *a priori* due to the fact that even the criteria of the classification are constructed and developed during the automatic reasoning process. This is possible because of the very strong generalisation mechanism included (or built in) the grammar parsing process. Owing to formal, powerful technologies for the automatic parsing of all linguistic formulas (describing actual images), we can recommend mathematical linguistic technology as the most powerful technology for any generalisation.

The only problem is to properly adjust the terms and methods of formal grammars and artificial languages to their application to images (e.g. languages for computer programming rather than strings of symbols, which are the form of natural languages and even most artificial ones). The problem is very well known to specialists but, for the completeness of our presentation, let us explain some fundamental ideas.

When we try to build a language for the description of images we must start with fundamental definitions of elements belonging to the suitable graph grammar. Let us assume that we must build a grammar for the description of a class of landscape, similar to the image presented on Fig. 7.5.

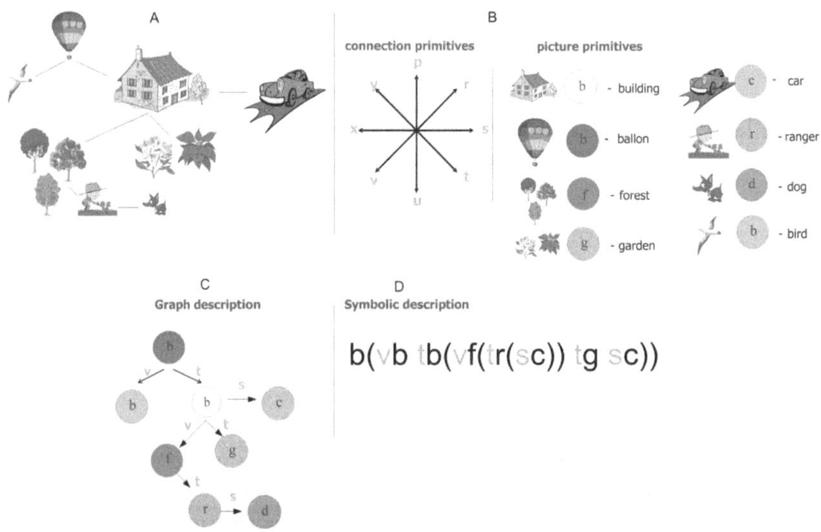

Fig. 7.5. Image for syntactic description. A) Analysed scene, B) Elements of vocabulary used, C) Symbolic representation of the scene before its description in terms of graph-grammar, D) Conversion of a graph diagram of the image into its symbolic description

An analysis of the scene under consideration shows that we have some classes of graphic objects ('primitives') which can be built into the grammar as substantives (nouns). We also have some classes of relations between objects, which can be treated as the verbs of our grammar. So the vocabulary of the grammar for the images under consideration can be shown as in Fig. 7.5.B.

Using the proposed vocabulary, we can replace the landscape image with an equivalent scheme for the grammar, as shown on Fig. 7.5.C.

On the basis of such a symbolic description of the image under consideration, we can also use symbolic notations for elements of the vocabulary; for every image they obtain a representation in terms of terminal symbols belonging to the definition of the grammar used (see Fig. 7.5.D).

After a final description of the image, using elements of the selected (or, most typically, purpose-built) image description language, we must implement the cognitive resonance concept. This is, of course, the most difficult part of the whole task. During the cognitive resonance, we must generate a hypothesis about the semantic meaning of the image under consideration and we must have an effective algorithm for its on-line verification. Both of these activities are performed by the parser of the grammar used. The hypothesis generation is connected with the use of a selected production (mappings included in the formal description of the grammar). The hypothesis generation process depends to a great extent on the medical problem. The hypothesis is verified by the incessant comparison of selected features of the image with expectations taken from the source of knowledge (mostly a medical doctor's experience based on his or her previous visual expertise).

The main idea of cognitive resonance is based on the iterative performance of the following steps. Let us assume that a semantic linguistic description of an image is written in the usual form of a string of terminal symbols (denoting for example a pattern in the form of the following text "medicalunderstandingbasedoncognitiveanalysis"):

μεδιχαλυνδερστανδινγβασεδονχογνιτιϖεαναλψσισ

We use Greek symbols as is traditional in mathematical linguistics, to show that a man does not need to understand symbols produced by the linguistic processor, it is enough if the parser can manage them.

Now the parsing process begins. Let us assume that **working hypothesis number 1** about the meaning of this image leads to the assumption that the image must include at least one pattern (e.g. "recognition"):

ρεχογνιτιον

The parser starts the process of searching through all strings of terminal symbols describing (in terms of the used language) important semantic features of the analysed image. The searching process fails, which means that the strength of working hypothesis no 1 decreases. Another working hypothesis leads to the assumption that the image must include at least one pattern ("cognitive"):

χογνιτιϖε

This pattern can be found in the analysed string:

μεδιχαλυνδερστανδινγβασεδονχογνιτιϖεαναλψσισ
χογνιτιϖε

which means that our working hypothesis no 2 can now be considered more probable. But we are still not quite sure wh ether the hypothesis is true or not as for its full validation it is necessary to also test other assumptions taken from this hypothesis and from all other hypotheses.

The description of cognitive resonance presented here is, of course, highly simplified. In fact, the set of methods and formulas used by the real parser designed by us especially for this work is a lot more complicated!That one will be shown in chapter 8 applied to practical examples.

7.4. Types of languages used in the syntactic approach to image description problems

This subsection will present definitions of basic types of image languages from the group of sequence, tree and graph grammars suitable for image recognition. For such languages, we will also present the definitions of syntactic analyzers which support recognizing elements of image descriptions defined using grammatical formalisms.

Definition 7.1. Attributive grammar [55]

An attributive grammar is defined as the quadruple $G = (V_n, V_t, SP, STS)$; where V_n, V_t represent finite sets of non-terminal and terminal symbols, STS is the grammar start symbol and the SP is a production set consisting of two parts: a syntactic rule and a semantic rule.

The syntactic rules have the form of: $X \rightarrow a$, for $X \in V_n$ and $a \in V_n \cup V_t$

On the other hand, the semantic rules are given in the following form:

$$Y_1 = f_1(X_{11}, X_{12},..., X_{1n1}, Y_1,..., Y_n), Y_2 = f_2(X_{21}, X_{22},..., X_{2n2}, Y_1,..., Y_n), ...$$

$$Y_n = f_n(X_{n1}, X_{n2},..., X_{nnn}, Y_1,..., Y_n)$$

where X_{ij} $(1 \leq i \leq n,\ 1 \leq j \leq n_i)$ are attributes of terminal or non-terminal symbols, f_i $(1 \leq i \leq n)$ are the assigned functions or appropriately defined semantic procedures; and Y_i $(1 \leq i \leq n)$ are attributes or defined variables employed in semantic actions.

Definition 7.2. A context-free grammar [55] is a grammar whose productions have the form: $A \rightarrow \gamma$, where $A \in \Sigma_N$, $\gamma \in \Sigma^+$

i.e. a non-terminal A is replaced by a non-empty γ sequence made of any combination of terminal and non-terminal symbols.

Definition 7.3. A context-free grammar $G = (V_N, V_T, SP, STS)$ is an LR(k)-type grammar (for $k \geq 0$) if, for each derivation step of forms:

$$STS \Rightarrow^R \mu A\omega \Rightarrow \mu\chi\omega,\ \mu \in V^*,\ \omega \in V_T^*,\ A \rightarrow \chi \in SP$$
$$STS \Rightarrow^R \mu' B\omega' \Rightarrow \mu'\gamma\omega',\ \mu' \in V^*,\ \omega' \in V_T^*,\ B \rightarrow \gamma \in SP$$

the condition $(|\mu\chi| + k): \mu\chi\omega = (|\mu'\gamma| + k): \mu'\gamma\omega'$ implies that: $\mu = \mu', A = B, \chi = \gamma$

where: $\Rightarrow^R$ denotes the right-hand derivation (right-hand derivation or a derivation step) in the grammar, i.e. in each new step, a new text string is derived from the rightmost non-terminal symbol.

$V = V_T \cup V_N$, $V^* = \{\mu: \mu = x_1x_2...x_n, n \geq 1, x_i \in V \text{ for } i = 1...n\} \cup \lambda$ (λ is an empty symbol)

$V_T^* = \{\omega: \omega = y_1y_2...y_m, m \geq 1, y_i \in V_T \text{ for } i=1...m\} \cup \lambda$,

$$k : w = \begin{cases} w \ \ when \ |w| < k \\ \alpha, \ when \ \omega = \alpha\gamma \ and \ |\alpha| = k \end{cases}$$

To analyze linguistic elements described by context-free grammars of the LR(k) type, LR(k) automata are used. Below, we will define the simplest class of them, i.e. LR(1) automaton.

Definition 7.4. An LR(1)-class automaton (or LR(1)) automaton for grammar G is the sequence:

$$LRA\ (G) = (Q, V_n, V_t, SP, q_0, \ next, reduce)$$

where: Q is a finite nonempty set of automaton states, V_n, V_t are finite sets of non-terminal and terminal symbols, SP is a production set, and $q_0 \in Q$ is the initial automaton state.

The function of the next state, *next,* is determined as:

$$next\colon\ Q \times (V_n \cup V_t \cup \{\$\})^* \rightarrow Q \cup \{stop\}$$

and satisfies the following conditions (symbol $is a limiter of the input sequence):

1. *next*(q, λ) = q
2. *next*(q, αx) = next(next(q, α), x)

The reduction function *reduce* is determined as:

$$reduce\colon\ Q \times (V_n \cup V_t \cup \{\$\})^* \rightarrow 2^{SP}$$

LR(1)-type automata belong to the group of reduction analysers, controlled by a steering table. The automaton operation is determined by two functions describing the analyser current state and defined in order to carry out a complete reduction analysis. These functions are: *action procedure* and *goto*.

The syntactic analysis starts with the initial automaton configuration, i.e. the application of the *action procedure* defined for the q_0 initial state and the first input sequence symbol.

A detailed description of the operating rules of reduction analyzers is presented in the following publication: [55].

Another interesting proposal in the field of structural analysis with the use of sequence languages are Languages of Shape Feature Description [55] which allow a somewhat more general analysis to be conducted based on the changes in so-called sinquads, i.e. distinguished directions in the space. Such languages are analyzed using multiple-input sequential transducers.

Definition 7.5. A multiple-input sequential transducer is a quintuple defined in the following way:

$$ST=(Q, \Sigma_T, \Delta, \delta, Q_0)$$

Where: Q- finite set of states, Σ_T- finite set of input symbols (terminals), Δ- finite set of output symbols, $Q_0 \subset Q$- set of initial states, δ-transition function defined as: $\delta\colon Q x \Sigma^*_T \longrightarrow Q x \Delta^*$

The notation $\delta(q,\gamma) = (q,\eta)$ means that after reading the input sequence $\gamma \in \Sigma^*_T$, the transducer moves from state q to q' and writes the $\eta \in \Delta^*$ sequence at the output. For the input sequence of $\gamma \in \Sigma^*_T$ terminal symbols, the sequence $\eta = ST(\gamma)$ is the output text string from the transducer if and only if there are the following sequences:

$$\gamma_1,\ldots,\gamma_k \in \Sigma^*{}_T\ ,\ \eta_1,\ldots,\eta_k \in \Delta^*\ ,\ q_1,\ldots,q_k \in Q$$

Satisfying the following conditions:

1. $\gamma = \gamma_1,\ldots,\gamma_k$,
2. $\eta = \eta_1,\ldots,\eta_k$,
3. $\delta(q_i, \gamma_{i+1}) = (q_{i+1}, \eta_{i+1})$ for i = 0, 1,..., k–1, $q_0 \in Q_0$.

An analysis with the use of sequential transducers is extremely effective when a description of the looked-for lesions is introduced in the form of languages describing shape features. This is especially important in diagnosing structures of particularly complex morphology.

Definition 7.6. Expansive G_{edt} tree grammar generating trees with a directed and labelled edge, i.e. EDT trees. It is defined as a set of five other sets defined as follows [19]:

$$G_{edt} = (\Sigma, \Gamma, r, P, Z)$$

where Σ is a set of terminal and non-terminal vertex labels, r is a function assigning to the tree vertex the number of its successors (children), Z is a finite set of start trees, Γ is a set of edge labels and P is a production set of the following form:

$$A \rightarrow a(\tau_1 A_1 \ \tau_2 A_2 ... \ \tau_{r(a)} A_{r(a)})$$

where: A_1, A_2 ... $A_{r(a)}$ are non-terminal vertexes while 'a' is a terminal vertex; $\tau_1, \tau_2 ... \tau_{r(a)}$ are edge labels.

The right-hand side of the production $a(\tau_1 A_1, \tau_2 A_2 ..... \tau_{r(a)} A_{r(a)})$ denotes an EDT tree written in the parentheses form. The tree has a root and r(a) successor leafs labelled A_1, A_2 .... $A_{r(a)}$, connected to the root by means of r(a) edges labelled as a τ_1, $\tau_2 ..... \tau_{r(a)}$ respectively and directed from the root to the leaves.

Definition 7.7. An A_{EDT} automaton with the output above a set of vertex labels $\Sigma_T = \{a_1, a_2, ... a_n\}$ and a set of edge labels Γ, which recognizes EDT trees, represents an (n +2) element set defined as follows:

$$A_{EDT} = (Q, \delta_1, ..., \delta_n, F), \text{ where:}$$

Q – is the finite set of states

δ_k – is a transition function defined as: $\delta_k : (\Gamma Q)^{r(ak)} \rightarrow Q \times N \ \{k = 1,...,n\}$

for $a_k \in \Sigma_T$, N – the set of natural numbers, $\Gamma Q = \{\tau A \mid \tau \in \Gamma, A \in Q\}$

$F \subseteq Q$ – the set of final states

Definition 7.8. An expansive graph grammar $\mathbf{G_{exp}}$ generating EDG graphs (Edge Directed Graphs) is the following ordered five:

$$G_{exp} = (N, \Sigma, \Gamma, P, S), \text{ where:}$$

N – a set of non-terminal peak labels,

Σ – a set of terminal peak labels,

Γ – a set of edge labels,

S – stands for the start symbol

P –a finite production set of one of two forms:

1. the reduced form: $A \rightarrow a$, $A \in N$, $a \in \Sigma$
2. the expansive form: $A \rightarrow a x_1 B_1 x_2 B_2^{e2} ... x_r B_r^{er}$, where: $a \in \Sigma$, $A, B_i \in N$, $x_i \in \Gamma$ (I = 1,...r), $e_i \in \{*, \lambda\}$ are the location operators

Definition 7.9. The name of G_{edNLC} (edge-labelled directed Node-Label Controlled graph) grammar refers to the set of five elements defined as follows [19, 23]:

$$G_{edNLC} = (\Sigma, \Delta, \Gamma, P, Z), \text{ where:}$$

- Σ is a finite, non-empty set of node labels. These labels denote additional nodes in the graphs that are entered as temporary during the syntax analysis.
- Δ (a subset of Σ) is a set of terminal (i.e. end-marking) node labels. These labels describe the terminal elements of the modelled structure.
- Γ is a finite, non-empty set of edge labels. This set makes it possible to define spatial relations occurring between the individual sections approximating the recognised elements.
- P is a finite production set in the form of (l, D, C), where $l \in \Sigma$, and D is an EDG graph. These productions define the graph-based language describing potential image cases.
- $C : \Gamma \times \{in, out\} \rightarrow 2^{\Sigma \times \Sigma \times \Gamma \times \{in, out\}}$ is an embedding transformation defining the manner of connecting old and new nodes during the syntactic analysis conducted.
- Z is the start graph, which is used to begin the process of generation of all graph-based forms for analysed images

Detailed descriptions of methods for performing a structural analysis using graph grammars are presented in publications including: [19, 49], so we will not describe them again here.

8. Image understanding methods applied to medical diagnostics

This chapter presents the practical operation of methods, algorithms and techniques described in previous ones. They will be presented using two selected examples. In previous papers and books (for example [34, 36, 37, 38, 39, 55]), we showed the applicability and proved the usefulness of the *automatic understanding* technology in some medical applications (e.g. pancreatic cancer or ureter stenoses), but all such examples were related to the organs presented in medical images as singular, convex, two-dimensional shapes. In this book, we try to extend the evaluation of the considered technologies to cover more complicated medical images. Specifically, we will present and discuss a new technique of computer-aided analysis and recognition of pathological wrist bone lesions. In this application, the *automatic understanding* technology must prove its utility for a complex anatomical structure (the hand), formed of many separate elements (wrist bones), where the pathologies considered can be represented not only by deformations of the forms, dimensions and shapes of particular selected bones, but can also be expressed in pathological relationships between individual bones. This problem is much more interesting from the scientific point of view, because *automatic understanding* is much more complicated when it is based on relationships between elements instead of analyzing one particular morphological element itself.

In this chapter we will also try to show and evaluate the applicability of the *automatic understanding* technology to modern 3D medical imaging. This type of imaging is now very "fashionable", for very important reasons. Anatomical structures are always three dimensional, which fact should be taken into account in every medical examination. When we record and evaluate only traditional 2D medical images, we can lose some important information. Therefore the progress in medical imaging is now closely connected with the elaboration and development of many new methods for the 3D reconstruction of medical structures. Such reconstructions can be produced on the basis of sequences of many 2D slides (for example in a CT of the brain). Thanks to computer visualization methods, such 3D reconstructions can be viewed from many points of view, close-up or from a distance, they can be rendered on the surface, or transparent and allowing the inner parts to be penetrated as well, they can be rotated in any direction and so on.

Automatic understanding methods can be particularly useful for computer aided medical diagnostics based on 3D imaging, because such imaging is always very nice to look at, but is in fact very hard to interpret precisely, especially in quantitative terms. We can say that physicians can see more on modern 3D visualizations of medical structures, but they understand less than from traditional 2D imaging. For this reason, our *automatic understanding* methods must also be tested with regard to tasks connected with assessing images obtained by means of 3D medical imaging. We will show an example of this in this book, using spatial reconstruction CT images of coronary vessels.

M.R. Ogiela and R. Tadeusiewicz: *Image understanding methods applied to medical diagnostics,* Studies in Computational Intelligence (SCI) **84**, 171–201 (2007)
www.springerlink.com

As mentioned above, we must first describe the images considered using AI graph-based linguistic formalisms. This will prove that our method uses AI techniques and mathematical linguistics which support the automatic evaluation and analysis of the structure of the said bones based on radiological images of the hand, and making a semantic description of spatial visualizations of coronary vessels. All details will be explained and presented in the following sections.

8.1. Graph image language techniques supporting cognitive interpretations of radiological hand images

The progress in soft-computing techniques, based on analyses which use graph image grammars, has had a significant impact on the development of medical information systems: they enable interpreting the meaning of some diagnostic image classes. The use of these techniques allowed using information systems for an in-depth semantic analysis aimed at formulating diagnostic recommendations and supporting the tasks associated with automatic medical diagnostics. In the field of image analysis where advanced techniques are used, the structural methods of applying graph and tree formalisms became crucial – for example, in the form of IE graphs (Indexed Edge-unambiguous) defined by ETPL(k)-type grammars (Embedding Transformation Preserved Production Ordered, k-left Nodes unambiguous) [19]. Such grammars allow us to describe complicated and multi-object image structures (including medical ones) and also as to interpret their meaning by executing semantic tasks. What is extremely important is that an analysis using graph image languages has a polygonal (square) complexity, which makes it very effective not only due to the significant descriptive power of graph languages, but also due to the speed at which the analysis is conducted.

Simpler classes of structural methods had been used earlier for semantic task analyses and for interpreting some medical images – in particular, those originating from examinations of the abdominal cavity structure [55]. However, these studies, presented in this chapter of the book, were based on the use of sequence languages, enabling an intelligent analysis of images that depicted individual structures or objects to be analyzed. In this chapter we will present an entirely new approach to the use of graph image languages supporting the tasks of interpreting and diagnosing radiographs. These types of images, due to their varied structure, are an example of a deeper, more complex analysis task. It is also worthwhile noting that the actual use of linguistic methods, enriched with semantic formalisms, can lead to a computer medical understanding of the meaning of recognized images. This is because there are a number of similarities between the operation of semantic analyzers used in such methods and the model of human visual perception [1, 55]. The main mechanism here is the stage of cognitive resonance, which means looking for coincidences between the expectations concerning the recorded cases and their actual features. As a result, these methods gain in importance and can be used on a wider scale, thus increasing the significance of the diagnostic interpretation of selected image classes. As such tasks are more and more frequently executed by specialised information systems, the development of such methods significantly contributes to the development of intelligent diagnostic systems and reasoning modules that can be integrated with PACS (Picture Archiving and Communication Systems).

The proposed structural AI techniques not only support the perception analysis of many images for diagnostic purposes, but more and more frequently they can also be used to create intelligent medical IT systems, supporting the medical diagnosis by means of intelligent searches in big medical databases [38]. Such systems are designed for different meaning and interpretation tasks dedicated to various medical data types, while their operation is based on the use of advanced AI techniques generally referred to as 'soft computing'.

The algorithms which describe the graph grammar, presented later in this chapter, expand the traditional methods of computer-aided analysis through the interpretation opportunities for supporting medical diagnostics. Additionally, semantic information facilitates using these techniques in tasks of semantically oriented searching for some specific disease cases in medical image databases. In practice, such tasks were difficult and sometimes even impossible to implement due to difficulties in creating indexing keys that describe image semantics [18, 38]. Expanding analytical possibilities by interpreting the meaning allows us to find answers to questions concerning the medical meaning of the analyzed image, semantic information specified by the features of the examined image and classification possibilities of disease entities based on lesions in the image.

Opportunities for the computer interpretation of selected images, based on the methodology of automatic medical image understanding introduced by the authors, were created due to the introduction of an original relational description of individual palm (wrist) bones and selected elements or the entire 3D structure of the coronary vascular tree. This description has been built with the use of graph linguistic formalisms already applied in artificial intelligence. These were, however, developed and adjusted to the needs of automatic medical image understanding in earlier works of the authors, as specified in the references section of this book. The research described in this chapter has demonstrated that specialist linguistic tools such as expansive graph grammars and EDT-label graphs are particularly well-suited for the purpose of palm (wrist) bone diagnostics. Defining a graph image language adjusted to the specific features of the scientific problem described here supported a semantic description of correct palm bone structures (with consideration to idiosyncratic features). It also supported the interpretation of images showing some in-born lesions, such as additional bones; or acquired lesions such as their incorrect junctions resulting from injuries and synostoses.

The analysis of images conducted in this chapter will go in the direction mapped out by the questions formulated. Its objective will be, in particular, to present and evaluate the possibilities of expansive graph grammar application for the recognition and the intelligent meaning analysis of radiographs of wrist ligaments and bones. In our research we defined effective, syntactic analyzer algorithms for graphs describing both cases of morphological elements falling within physiological norms, and selected cases of diseases showing their symptoms as visible irregularities on analyzed radiographs. The appropriateness of the cognitive analysis of such structures using computer semantic analysis methods has been dictated, among others, by the following factors:

1. A 2D image analysis of most objects under consideration is more difficult than the typical image analysis since some details are blurred in hand images as a result of bones overlapping each other. This can lead to the apparent disappearance of some bones, hidden behind other ones and the algorithm must 'guess' the form of the bone and its relation to the other elements in the image.
2. Sometimes one can find additional bones or bone decrements on a hand image, not described a priori by anatomical maps. Such phenomena can be caused by joints which do not exceed physiological norms and belong to normal individual differences between people.
3. Images can display fractures and displacements, caused by injuries and other pathological processes.

A cognitive analysis of hand images may supply a lot of significant information of diagnostic and therapeutic importance. This is true not only for traumas and diseases solely in the wrist area. Changes of bone morphology may point to the existence of a number of in-born pathological lesions, but they can also suggest acquired disease lesions demonstrating, for example, metabolic disorders. Of course, the above-listed factors can, in various combinations, contribute to deformations caused by mechanical injuries. The diagnosis of the upper limb differential allows us also to recognize and, later, to treat a number of soft-tissue diseases. Such cases, however, shall not be considered at this stage of the research.

The research described in this chapter has focused primarily on the analysis of the number and spatial relations between individual wrist bones. An intelligent interpretation of the analyzed cases can enable the identification of lesions such as the occurrence of *os centrale* or other additional wrist bones. It may also point to a lack of or to lesions in the shape of scaphoid or capitate bones as well as their synostoses with other wrist parts. Along with the progress in the development of research and syntactic image recognition techniques, analyses will become increasingly more complex. This means that more and more subtle irregularities in the number, structure and mutual location of bones in the wrist will be detected.

8.1.1. Characteristics of the analyzed data

The analysis of hand bone correctness has been based on examples from about a dozen selected hand X-rays, obtained both in the anterio-posterior (AP) and posterio-anterior (PA) projections.

It should be noted that the complete set of analyzed radiographs initially included about 50 real images of which some presented correct structures (falling within the anatomical and physiological norms with regards to their location, mobility and the number of wrist bones) that originated from radiological screening research. Some images were selected since they revealed pathologies that were of interest to us. The latter, at the current stage of conceptual development (but not yet an efficiency analysis) of the syntactic method of analyzing wrist bone pathology were not obtained by the authors but were taken from diagnostic atlases [9]. Owing to this, the morphology description as well as the diagnostic classification of these images can be considered as certain and unquestioned. Moreover, owing to the use of these very examples, every reader can check the operation of methods proposed by us by referring to the same, known and commonly available data.

We would like to emphasize that the authors realize the need to conduct significant verification and validation of new algorithms on possibly large sets of original data. This is why after preparing and optimizing this method, wider empirical research will be conducted on its properties and limitations, based on original images from a number of orthopedic clinics. In the future, the analysis of results from many concrete examples will allow us to collect and present credible statistics showing the efficiency of a syntactic analysis method used as a tool for the cognitive analysis of this form of medical images. This, however, will take place later and will be the subject of a separate publication. This is due to the fact that this chapter is aimed at purely presenting the methods proposed by us and promoting their use, but not at assessing them. For this reason this chapter contains no analysis of the statistical results and the information quoted in it should be treated solely as examples and rough data.

The two described medical image subsets played different roles during examinations whose results are presented in this chapter. The correct images constituted the material that allowed us to define the necessary linguistic mechanisms in the form of a graph. This constituted the basis for creating an appropriate expansive grammar defining the set of possible wrist bone cases as well as their mutual relations, falling within physiological norms. Owing to a codification of the physiological norm in the form of basic rules of the analyzed grammar, an effect was achieved such that the syntax analysis of all generated descriptions for new analyzed images became the sufficient tool to obtain answers. This applied whether the case analyzed fell within the norms accepted and specifying a correct hand image, or whether we were dealing with some form of a pathology.

On the other hand, selected cases of pathological images allowed us to add to the generated grammar a set of rules introducing some special patterns of typical morphological irregularities. Owing to the inclusion of these incorrect situations in the categories of additional grammar rules (going beyond physiological frameworks), it has also become possible to recognize some additional bones that can occur on X-ray images of an irregular wrist. A grammar analysis of the wrist bone morphology also enables us to diagnose and correctly interpret a reduction in their number, for example as a result of neighboring bone synostosis. The diagram showing the possible occurrence of additional bones, initially taken into consideration in the research, is shown in Figure 8.1. However, due to the large number of such potentially possible irregularities and due to the negligible fraction of the population in which some of them were recorded, further analysis issues have been narrowed down only to objects marked with grey areas in Figure 8.1. Fields marked grey in the figure show the most frequent places in which additional bones of closer series, and those located between the closer and further wrist series, cover a set of about 90% of the most frequent images of pathologically formed wrists.

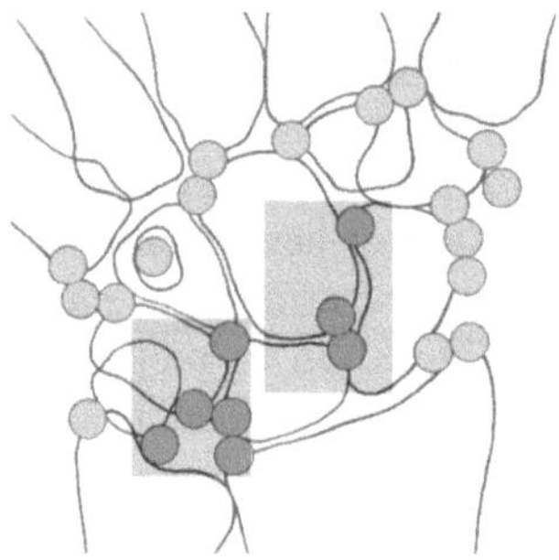

Fig. 8.1. The location and number of possible additional wrist and hand bones. Grey areas stand for additional bones of closer hand bone series recognizable by the grammar defined in this chapter

Real examples of images showing pathological lesions in the form of wrist bone dislocation, necrosis, and fusion are shown on Figure 8.2. Such irregularities are to be detected and interpreted correctly by the syntactic image recognition method described in this chapter.

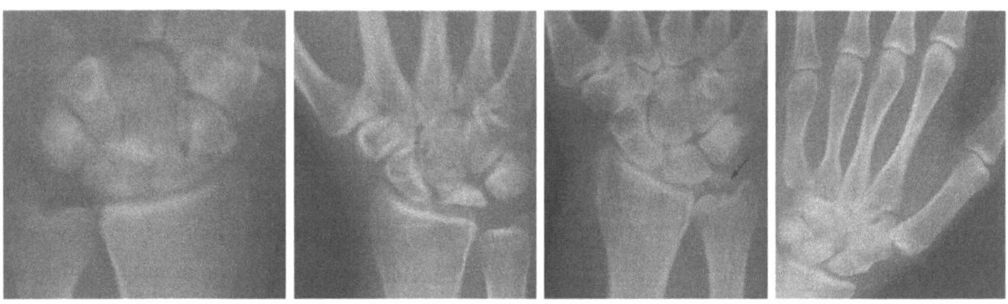

Fig. 8.2. A) An image showing lesions in the form of a lunate dislocation. B) A case of avascular necrosis of the lunate (Kienbock's disease). C) An image showing the calcification (arrow) in the triangular region of the wrist. D) The fusion of the scaphoid with the distal row of carpal bones

Let us point out one methodological remark here. As was proven during the research process, only a few typical images are enough for establishing all the necessary grammar rules. This means that even a small size of the research sample can give the necessary outcome for the initial specification of a certain model pattern, for which image languages have been defined. Such languages, however, enable a generalization of the pattern classification and, as a result, allow us to effectively recognize a practically unlimited number of new cases, similar (in some way) to elements registered during the formation of grammar rules. Such a generalizing property is, of course, a characteristic feature of all linguistic formalisms with a high generation capacity, i.e. which allow us to describe complicated shapes or relations with the use of a small number of language rules [55]. This also results from the fact that linguistic mechanisms, defining a given language, in reality define a set containing a lot more objects than the samples used to build it. This is also the case with applying graph grammar to hand image analyses: it facilitates defining the grammar *a priori* used to recognize the grammar.

A correct definition of graphs spinning metacarpal bones and finger bones (phalanx) has been made with EDG type graphs (graphs with directed nodes and with labeled nodes and edges) [50].

All images analyzed here were, before their analysis, subjected to pre-processing [3, 26, 55] aimed at showing bone contours of the closer and further hand bone series and identifying /*labeling*/ them, which later facilitates a search of the spanned graph with a selected width analysis technique.

In order to obtain a wrist bone description in the form of a graph it is necessary to conduct pre-processing operations first. These result in separating individual parts of wrist structures. Among such operations. the most important are the wrist image segmentation and the operation of spanning the graph on the closer and further wrist bones. To extract individual bones and separate their contours on the examined X-ray images, we tried to use the histogram programming algorithm and the method of hand structure separation as described in paper [34, 46]. However, owing to this, the results obtained by simple thresholding were not completely satisfactory, and due to the dedicated character of the second specified method, we later resorted to a semi-automatic algorithm for tracing individual bone contours. Originally this algorithm was designed for an entirely different purpose, i.e. for the extraction of pancreatic duct edges [27]. Research has demonstrated that after specifying starting points for the search of edges of every bone, it was possible to find their contours (Figure 8.3) even if structures overlapped. During the analysis for overlapping bones it is necessary to mix the segmentation results obtained from analyses made sequentially on separately binarized neighboring bones.

After the initial definition of the individual object edges, images underwent operations to make up for losses (for example by means of closing contours morphologically) and to label them by filling each bone contour. In the case of the radial bone and the ulnar bone as well as the closer bones of the metacarpus, which are also taken into consideration during the design of a graph description, only those articular parts were taken into consideration whose edges were defined to lie at the level of necks (narrowings other than the acetabulum) of individual bones.

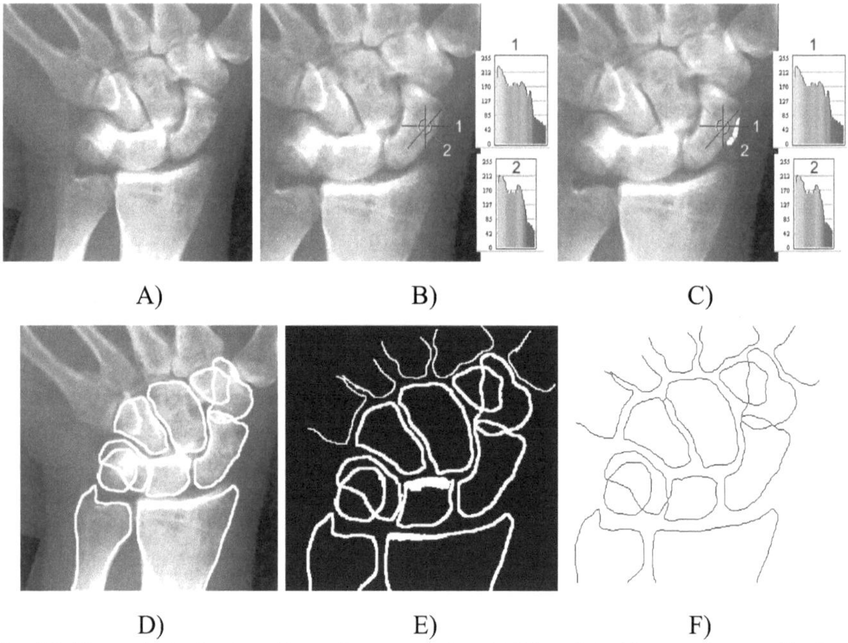

Fig. 8.3. The method of wrist radiograph segmentation. A) The original image after equalization. B, C) The "Star-section" method of wrist bone thresholding. Histograms showing segmentation levels are visible. D) The result of wrist bone segmentation. E) The image after binarization, morphological contour closing and median filtration. F) Wrist bone contours obtained using Pavlidis thinning algorithm

Following this, based on indexing labels, individual bones and their centers of gravity were determined on images thus prepared and binarized. They formed the spanning points for the graph representation introduced. Mutual topological relations between individual elements were introduced at the stage of constructing a linguistic representation and they were arbitrarily defined as shown in Figure 8.4. It is worth emphasizing, however, that the values of labels defining these relations were determined empirically using available data so as to enable the differentiation of possible individual bone locations and clearly determining their mutual location or possible dislocations. In order to avoid representational ambiguity obtained with such labels, for images showing the hand structures slightly twisted, prior to starting labeling the edges of a graph spanned on gravity centers of individual bones, it was rotated in such a way that the first edge coming out of the radial bone to the ulnar bone (i.e. the root of graph number 1, representing the radial bone to peak numbered 2, representing the ulnar bone) received a vertical orientation label. Such an operation is possible since it does not change any mutual relations between bones. At the same time it makes the introduced representation more universal, independent of the possible twisting of the hand in the image. The starting point for the analysis is, in every case, the peak labeling of the radial bone. This is where facilitation matters. The graph representation was introduced to images executed in the PA projection of the left wrist. In the case of the bones in the right wrist, the representation is obtained by making a mirror vertical reflection at the stage of initial analysis.

8.1.2. A syntactic description of wrist radiographs

In order to introduce a graph representation, it is necessary to define both the graphic elements (so called primitives, which have to be recognized automatically during the first step of the classification process) and the spatial relations between the recognized objects. In order to obtain a spinning graph (a formal description of the examined bones) from the analyzed image, it is necessary first to identify and label all the bones of the closer and further wrist series: their analysis is important from the diagnostic point of view. Next, it is necessary to specify spatial relations in accordance with the accepted order (Figure 8.4).

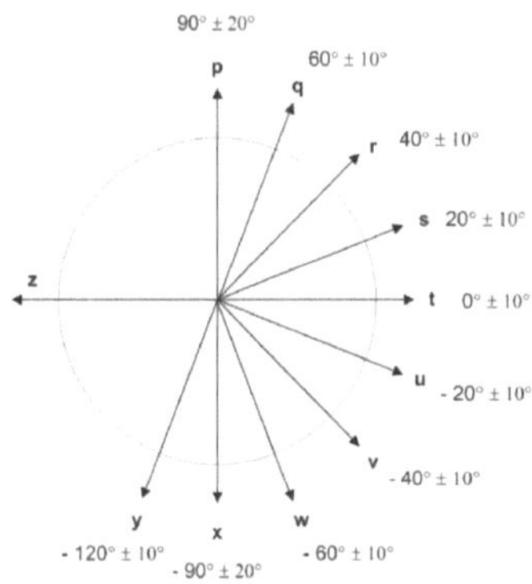

Fig. 8.4. Graph spatial relationships

The scheme described is a simplified one, because on X-ray photographs obtained in real life, instead of this regular pattern one can find a very complicated and irregular system of wrist bone forms and locations, necessitating a proper adjustment of the theoretical graph description to real X-ray images. In fact, a real representation of the three-dimensional system of hand bones onto a 2D plane may cause difficulties in such a process. This is due to the fact that sometimes some details become blurred or even disappear. In the case of the hand skeleton, this phenomenon can be observed, for example, for the trapezoid bone, which disappears hidden under the trapezium and capitate bones or, in the case of the pisiform, hidden by the triquetrum bone. On the other hand, the scaphoid and the capitate bones overlap causing the limits between them to blur (they are shown differently, depending on the analyzed AP or PA projection) [9].

Bearing the above difficulties in mind, we should use a graph representing a correct bone system (spanned also on the metacarpal) for the analysis of the most common type of images. The sample image shown on Fig. 8.5 allows us to establish a graph that describes these hands in a very easy way. This is because the presented wrist has the correct structure, the position of the hand is properly adjusted and the hand of the patient is healthy, without any lesions or mechanical injuries (see Fig 8.5). This example proves that a graph description of images of the hand can be used to determine its form in correct cases as well as to diagnose various irregularities, as the exceptions from the accepted norm. In the case of the correct structure of the hand and a well-taken X-ray, it is also possible to identify all the primary components and the relations between them in accordance with previously accepted patterns. In the case of illnesses, some of them can be missing.

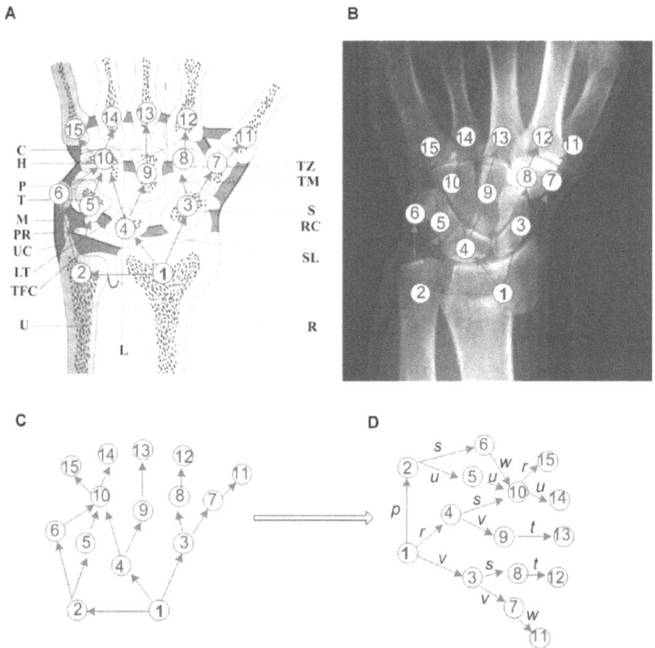

Fig. 8.5. The definition of an EDG graph describing the wrist skeleton. A) The anatomical scheme of a regular wrist (carpus) bone system with selected elements, which are necessary for the formal definition of the constitutive parts of a linguistic description based on the graph-grammar under consideration. B) A defined graph spanned on a real (correct) radiographic hand image. C) A graph extracted from the analyzed image. D) A graph in a form destined for analyzing with the graph grammar analyzer. In this graph, numbers denote nodes standing for neighboring wrist bones, while letters stand for the spatial relations between these bones (for easier analysis, the graph has been rotated clockwise by 90 degrees)

For the representation of the examined structures introduced in the form of EDG graphs [50], it is necessary to define an appropriate linguistic formalism, that is an appropriate graph grammar defining a language. The language is defined in such a way that it can be used to describe, without any ambiguities, every image representing a spatial system composed of elements similar to the wrist bone system. This way, we create a tool which describes all possible shapes and locations of wrist bones, both correct and pathological. The linguistic formalism that we propose in this chapter to execute the task of mirroring real medical image forms into graph formulas fit for computer processing consist in an expansive graph grammar [49, 55]. After defining such a grammar, every X-ray image will be converted into a linguistic formula built in accordance with the rules of that grammar. The effective parsing of that formula conducted by the computer, in accordance with the rules of the created grammar, will lead to an automatic assessment of image contents. This will make it possible, in particular, to determine whether the structure of the wrist falls within the norm or whether it exhibits pathological deviations.

8.1.3. The graph language describing the wrist structure

The above analysis shows that the key to the automatic interpretation of X-ray hand bone images considered in this chapter is an expansive graph grammar G_{exp} generating EDG graph, and defined below.

$$G_{exp} = (N, \Sigma, \Gamma, P, S),$$

where the following letters stand for:

- N – a set of non-terminal peak labels,
- Σ – a set of terminal peak labels,
- Γ – a set of edge labels,
- S – the start symbol,
- P – a finite production set.

In the research conducted, which is aimed at generating a linguistic description of the correct location and number of wrist bones, individual sets of the prepared grammar have been defined in the following way (labels consistent with Figure 8.5 and the names of individual bones on which graph nodes have been spanned).

Non-terminal set of peak labels N = {ST, ULNA SCAPHOID, LUNATE, TRIQUETRUM, PISIFORM, TRAPEZIUM, TRAPEZOID, CAPITATE, HAMATE, M1, M2, M3, M4, M5}.

Terminal set of peak labels Σ = {r, u s, l, t, p, tm, tz, c, h, m1, m2, m3, m4 m5}

Γ – edge label set presented in Figure 8.4.

Start symbol S = ST

P – is a finite production set presented in Figure 8.6.

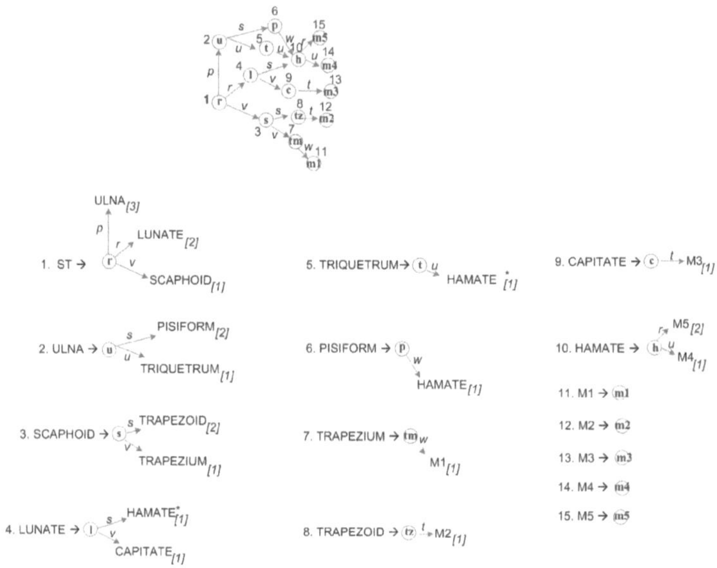

Fig. 8.6. A production/graph set introducing a representation of the correct structure and the number of bones in the wrist

The possibilities of describing image cases showing additional wrist bones can be obtained by enriching the above-presented set of rules introducing the formulas of the analyzed grammar to include productions defined in Figure 8.7. The set of non-terminal labels N will then also contain an additional peak label, 'Acc Bone', standing for the reasoning graph for the new object/bone appearing in the image (in the first series) and located in accordance with the labeled directions.

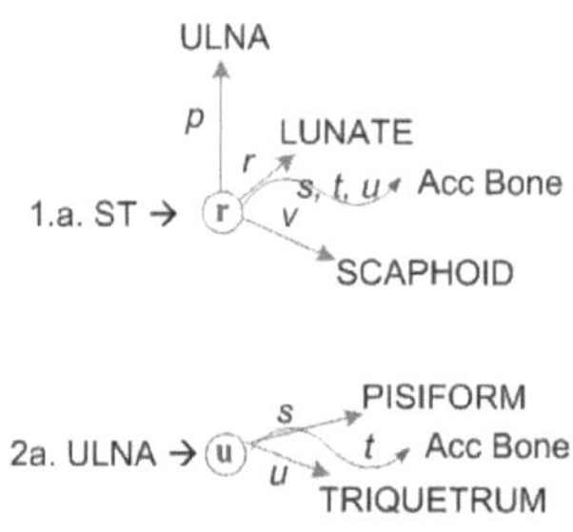

Fig. 8.7. A production set describing additional bones located in areas marked with circles on Figure 8.1. For simplification, peak and graph ordinals as well as graph location and operators were omitted from these productions

An image showing other forms of pathologies in the wrist image – synostoses or bone defects – can be recognized with the use of alternative rules specified in Figure 8.8. In this case an additional 'Fuss' peak appears and stands for the introduction of an additional bone, originating from the merger of two neighboring ones.

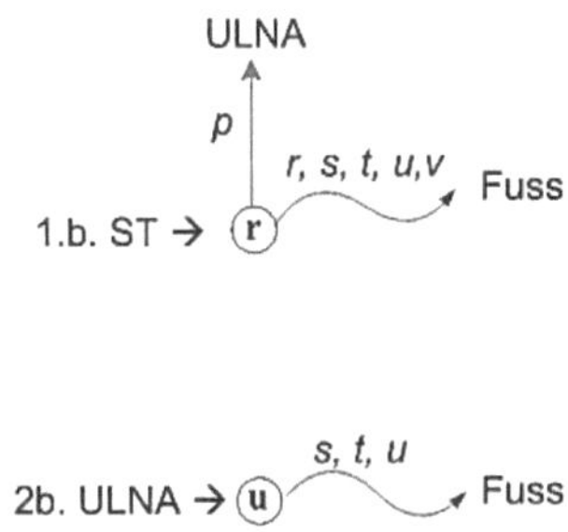

Fig. 8.8. A production set describing bone defects caused by bones fusing or by bone dislocation

8.1.4. Selected results

As a result of the conducted research, linguistic formalisms in the form of IE graphs [1, 51] were defined. Such graphs are a subset of EDG graph grammars [54]. These described both the radiographs of the regular hand bones and radiographs presenting some lesions falling within physiological norms, such as the appearance of additional bones or a reduction in their number. The presented methods were used for the computer analysis of selected radiograph sequences which originated both from radiological examinations and from specially selected and extremely rare cases, taken from books on radiology. All cases of the disappearance or appearance of objects important from the point of view of medical diagnostics were analyzed independently for their anterio-posterior and further posterio-anterior projections. The approach presented in this section also relates to changes in the number of bones and their location if they occur in a closer series or between the closer and further series. In subsequent research, these methods will also be adapted to analyze additional formations appearing in the metacarpus as a result of disease processes, in particular broken bones, incorrect synostoses and processes related to degenerative diseases (among others, the degenerative joint disease).

It should be emphasized that in the accepted methodology of structural (syntactic) image description, the key element is to define the grammar correctly so that it enables one to obtain a linguistic description of the foreseen images, both of correct and pathological forms of the analyzed anatomical structure (in this case, the wrist). Recognizing the structure of the examined image (wrist) therefore consists in a set of routine activities that can be fully automated. In our case, we decided to use a two-course syntax analyzer that first generates characteristic descriptions of nodes for the examined graphs and then conducts a generation analysis (top-down). As a result, sequences of grammar rule numbers are obtained as the output of the image analyzing system. These allow us to generate the analyzed graph description. Details of this kind of analysis can be found in [51]. However, it is worth emphasizing that the complexity of the structural analysis with the use of such grammars is multinomial. This means that the analyzing software can perform some activities very quickly, providing real-time support for decisions made by a physician watching archive images, for example in the PACS system.

The methods developed were aimed at building an automatic detection and semantic interpretation system for detected regularities as well as irregularities diagnosed in carpus bones. It is worth noting, however, that the test data set used to define output rules in the presented grammar was composed of only about 50 radiographs. Despite such an insignificant representation, and owing to the great descriptive and generation capacity of the graphs used, it is possible to classify practically any number of analyzed images. The initially assessed efficiency exceeds the 92% threshold. On the other hand, the appearance of difficult and ambiguous cases can be quickly considered by enriching grammar formalisms to include new reasoning rules (not considered before due to the lack of empirical data) and by specifying the meaning interpretation of such new cases. This is also the direction that will be followed in the research conducted.

The approach presented here is characterized by a certain universality while the obtained analysis results are independent of the hand's orientation. The research presented here so far relates to the analysis of radiographs obtained in the PA projection (both for the left and right hand). It turns out, however, that this stage of edge labeling for graphs spanned on individual bone parts allows us to obtain an independent analysis of results from the insignificant twisting of the hand. Should the whole image be rotated, it is also possible to obtain correct results provided that the initial analysis points are shown, i.e. the radial and the ulnar bones. The research conducted also demonstrates that only small modifications of the algorithm are necessary to analyze images in the AP projection. These are basically an analysis of a graph symmetric mirroring and the insignificant correction of a graph node location, brought about by a minor shifting of the centers of gravity that may occur in the consideration of such a projection. The automatic analysis could be hindered by cases including additional bones or defects that result in difficulties at the segmentation stage. However, the number of wrong diagnoses in such cases is very small and one must take into account the possibility of a manual interference and the manual pinpointing of the starting points for the constructed graph edges.

8.1.5. Conclusions concerning semantic analysis methods for wrist bones

This chapter presents a new approach to the intelligent, image-meaning analysis of wrist X-rays, making use of linguistic artificial intelligence methods in the form of graph image languages based on EDG grammars.

The use of such grammars represents an important step towards the use of structural graph methods in practical tasks of analysing complex multi-object images, i.e. wrist radiographs. This is an important expansion of previous research on the use of structural application methods for medical image analysis [10, 34, 36] that related primarily to single structures or organs and did not take into consideration the analysis of objects composed of many parts. Such structures include the wrist and hand bones. In their case, the difficulties with the analysis boil down to a context analysis taking into consideration the number and mutual topologies of individual parts rather than the classification of individual bones (easy to classify with methods used in this chapter or with contour pattern adjustment techniques). In this respect, the research presented seems to be valuable for utilitarian reasons since after an improvement of the methods presented here, they can be used in diagnostic practice.

These methods allow us not only to support the tasks of diagnosing acquired or inborn lesions as seen in the form of defects, morphology deformations or dislocations of wrist bones, but they are also aimed at making interpretations of the meaning of such images. This means that linguistic methods allow us to steer, in a meaningful way, the automatic computer interpretation of medical meaning in the pathological cases under examination. All this is possible because semantic information is gathered in the course of the syntactic analysis conducted. The application of structural methods can therefore significantly expand the opportunities offered by traditional medical information systems and medical diagnostic support systems. Moreover, such procedures could create semantic PACS system components that, in their operation, would support the semantic categorization and indexing of various diagnostic images, including those showing complex medical structures of organs. Meaning description, in the form of semantic records, can refer not only to the images of individual organs but also to spatial structures that depict mutual spatial relations between their elements (i.e. neighboring organs).

8.2. Picture grammars for classifying 3D coronary vessel visualizations

The successful development of a technique to be used for the automatic understanding of flat images encourages the development of similar methods for spatial representations of examined biological structures that can be provided by state-of-the-art imaging systems. The solutions presented in this study may pertain especially to the spatial visualization of coronary vessels, and these vessels will be used as examples in the detailed part of the study, yet both the very posing of the problem and the proposed method for its solution can be used more broadly.

Today's state-of-the-art methods of image diagnostics provide abundant and varied diagnostic and research material, as 3D visualizations are available for practically all human body structures and organs. They can illustrate the pathological lesions to a greater degree and more completely, assuming however that the physicians interpreting the image can understand well what they see and what it means. Clinical practice proves that, despite the frequent use of major computer-assisted diagnostic equipment, the visualizations (including the spatial reconstructions of specific body parts) obtained later undergo only a rough qualitative assessment by the physician diagnostician, with no in-depth semantic analysis. This is due to a number of reasons.

Firstly, the entire education system of physicians still predominantly uses flat images: they are presented in lectures and books as 2D and not 3D. Physicians have become accustomed to such images and can provide their diagnostic interpretations, while they find the 3D renderings – in fact closer to the actual anatomical or pathomorphological condition – less known if not 'exotic' and, consequently, harder to interpret.

Secondly, the progress in IT, electronics, and the development of research in the field of Medical Imaging make the evolution of visualization methods very fast: in fact, much faster than the process of gathering experience by the physicians who should expertly interpret those new visualizations. For that reason, it is often the case that a new method of medical visualization does present the essence of a medical problem, but the physician watching such a new visualization is unable to interpret it properly because, in simple words, there are so many things shown that he or she does not know what to look at. To make matters even worse, the aforementioned progress in the visualization technology still accelerates more and more, which means that by the time today's alumni become experienced masters in the field of interpreting certain state-of-the-art forms of medical visualization, these forms of visualization will have become dated and replaced by successive, even finer ones, which are again not in line with the experience acquired by the physicians.

Thirdly and lastly, there is something known as the spatial imagination. Some have it, others do not. The mutual relations between elements on a flat image can be interpreted correctly by anyone, while making correct conclusions referring to the interdependencies and relative placement of spatially perceived elements requires those special skills. This means that a certain proportion of physicians, and there are good reasons to believe that this can be quite a large proportion, will never be able to understand and correctly interpret the spatial co-dependences of the elements viewed. This deficiency will always limit the efficacy of their diagnostic reasoning, however suggestive and impressive the images displayed on the screens of ever finer 3D visualization systems: this effect has to be borne in mind.

These remarks prove that the actual progress in the practical application of 3D visualizations in medicine may depend on the progress in developing smart diagnostics support systems, making use of the automatic analysis and understanding of medical 3D images.

Due to the various meanings assigned to the term *understanding* and its crucial importance for this study, let us define that a certain computer-assisted interpretation of the 3D image examined meets the requirements of "automatic understanding" when the direct results of this interpretation include the 3D structure of the organ examined, the spatial relations between this structure and other organs and parts of the body, and what the consequences of this specific structure and relations are. Taking into account both diagnostic and therapeutic needs, we shall particularly require that the process of automatic understanding points to where, how, and with what consequences the pathological process has interfered with the natural (normal though differing between persons) 3D structure of the given organ. Using thus defined automatic understanding of 3D medical images, we can provide the physician with far more numerous and useful premises for therapeutic decisions than we would receive from the traditional paradigm of image recognition, which ends in the delivery of the decision (correct or not) stating the name of the diagnostic condition recognized and referring to an assumed – usually in an arbitrary manner – taxonomy of the diseases considered.

Naturally, the practical implementation of the postulate of understanding 3D medical visualization requires resorting to algorithms and information techniques far more advanced than those connected with the traditional automatic understanding and classification. Such, however, is the role of science that it must outpace the potential offered by the methods known and generally applied in pursuit of new approaches that better fulfill practical requirements: for that reason, in this study, we will deal with the construction of cognitive systems supporting the semantic analysis of 3D visualizations used in diagnostic systems.

8.2.1. The classification problem

In this section, we will show that graph formalisms based on IE graphs allow the semantic interpretation of irregularities visualized inn images obtained during diagnostic examinations of the heart muscle. The basis for the construction of 3D reconstructions of biological objects are visualizations obtained from helical CT scans. The semantic information obtained makes it possible to find a description of the structure focused on the semantics of various morphological forms of the visualized vessels from the point of view of the operation of coronary circulation and the blood supply of the heart muscle. Thanks to these, the analysis conducted allows a fast and – to a great efficiency – automated interpretation of the semantics of various morphological changes in the coronary vascular tree, and especially makes it possible to detect these stenoses in the lumen of the vessels that can cause critical decreases of the blood supply to extensive or especially important fragments of the heart muscle.

The problem tackled in this work is the semantic interpretation and an attempt at automatic understanding of a 3D structure of spatially visualized coronary vessels. At the initial analysis stage it was found that the problem is subject to numerous important limitations. These limitations result, among other things, from the serious obstacles encountered in the development of a universal standard, defining the model shape of the healthy or diseased organ that could possibly undergo typical recognition. Such difficulties were encountered already in the case of analyzing 2D images of various organs, however, the additional degree of freedom given by the transition from a 2D to a 3D visualization makes this question exceptionally intricate.

A certain level of repetitiveness and regularity is characteristic for the coronary vessels in different patients with various pathological forms observed on flat, i.e. 2D, images. The same images registered by a machine rendering 3D images (a helical CT scanner) feature a much greater number of visible details, which, however, also results in the increase of the number of both individual differences and those between various examinations of the same patient. Having considering these difficulties and the arguments quoted in the introduction to this chapter, a decision was made to apply the methods of automatic image understanding for the interpretation of the images considered, which consequently leads to their semantic descriptions. Thanks to such a posing of the problem, the diagnosis put forth (being naturally but a suggestion for the physician making the actual decision) will account for a greater number of factors and better use the available medical information. Additionally, it is worth pointing out that – even though this is not the main focus of the work presented here – the solution of problems related to the automatic production of intelligent (cognitive) descriptions of the 3D medical images in question may make a significant contribution to solving at least some of the problems connected with the smart archiving of this type of data and the finding of semantic image data meeting the semantic criteria delivered through sample image patterns in medical multimedia databases.

The above goals cannot be reached should the IT methodology applied be limited solely to the methods of automatic processing, analysis or even image recognition. The processed medical image may be more convenient for visual interpretation or easier for automatic analysis, yet this would not move the question of interpreting its meaning forward. Similarly, image analysis, providing the values of these or those parameters describing objects visible in the image as well as automatic recognition that allows their classification do not in fact answer the most fundamental questions asked by the physician. These are questions concerning the nature of the disease that the patient suffers from, the situation of the potentially dangerous stenoses and possible therapeutic suggestions, which, however, calls for the understanding of the content of the medical visualization, and not solely its formal analysis. What becomes necessary in such cases is the application of more advanced IT techniques, and particularly reaching for the so-called computational intelligence methods with generalization attributes. The application of the linguistic description, making use of special languages reaching into the semantic field of the patterns registered (also as images) opens the possibility of its understanding with methods derived from the parsing of appropriate grammars. The parsers suggested in this chapter (and their future, updated versions that are the subject of current research work) shall allow the conversion of an image description built around the language suggested into a description in semantic terms and shall make it possible to understand all the significant medical facts related to the image. The linguistic and cognitive methodology postulated in this chapter shall allow the creation of hybrid records at further stages of the analysis; such records will contain both the considered 3D images and their automatically generated cognitive descriptions containing the definition of their semantic properties.

Quite naturally, the path to finding appropriate languages, necessary for the description of the semantic aspect of the 3D medical visualization is long and complex. The description of important semantic aspects of the image may not be burdened with details that – from the point of view of understanding the contents of the image – are of secondary importance. This is why, besides the development of methods for the linguistic description of 3D images and the development of intelligent methods of using experts' experience and knowledge for acquiring the effect of cognitive resonance, of key importance for image understanding is the application of pre-processing methods and analysis of 3D medical visualizations adjusted to the specific features of this task. Hence, this work will also include finding such methods of extracting and describing medical image features that would ignore individual distinctive features characteristic for a given patient, while at the same time focusing on the exposition and the appropriate representation of morphological properties crucial for the understanding of pathologies presented in visualizations. Only well-selected elements of the description at the level of automatically identified elements of the visualization and their spatial relations may form the basis for the development of a language description that would later, at the parsing stage, support analyzing the semantics and detecting symptoms of the progressing medical condition. Elements of the description spatial mentioned above, treated as letters of the alphabet symbols, and the groundwork for the construction of specific language formulas, must be especially oriented towards discovering pathologic lesions: this will support not only locating those lesions but also interpreting their nature and, later, defining their medical significance.

The goal of this chapter, therefore, is to present the ways of taking the methodology [55] that has been developed earlier for the needs of automatic understanding of 2D medical visualizations to the level of 3D visualizations. The research will cover the potential of defining, in these visualizations, of elements describing the morphology of lesions and the possibility of applying the linguistic approach as well as cognitive image analysis for the description and modeling of spatial biomedical structures. The considerations will make reference especially to the 3D structure of the coronary vascular tree, which will be described with the use of graph-based languages of shape feature description [54]. The selection of such a linguistic technique results from the fact that – thanks to the application of advanced formalisms referring, *inter alia*, to the knowledge and experience of expert physicians – these languages make it possible to automatically identify places in the analyzed image that are crucial from the point of view of medical diagnostics, and after the definition of appropriate structural relations also support locating and defining the degree of advancement of lesions. Using such methods of computational intelligence greatly improves the ability to automatically interpret complex physiological and pathological processes unrolling in the visualized organ, at the same time supporting the semantic analysis that makes computer-assisted understanding of images possible. The methods proposed further in the chapter are oriented towards this type of tasks.

The proposal presented below may be perceived as a scientific contribution that contributes to further progress in diagnosing cardiovascular diseases. The problem embarked upon in this work may be considered significant due to the frequency of the practical use of identification of location of stenoses in coronary vessels in ischemia, being one of the most urgent medical problems of the early 21st century. Despite the huge progress in the equipment that allows obtaining a great variety of coronary vessels visualizations, and especially the latest achievements that support their 3D visualization, the progress in the automatic analysis of these images is highly limited, and most research is sill done manually by the operator or diagnostician. The technical solutions proposed do not aim at eliminating the physician from the diagnostic process; on the contrary, they should provide the physician with additional information to make him or her more efficient in discriminating obvious cases from ones that may require a more thorough consideration. A system for understanding 3D medical images may also facilitate interpreting especially complex and atypical cases, when even the physician's knowledge combined with experience may be insufficient for the diagnosis and defining the treatment strategy. Here, a system that offers an automatic semantic case assessment based on its 3D image may come in very handy, as it may, for example, make up for the spatial imagination that the given physician may lack. Furthermore, such an approach can also be applied to context-sensitive and semantic searches of databases to find medical spatial models showing changes in the morphology of coronary arteries in the semantic sense (i.e. the nature of the pathology and the treatment required) similar to the case under examination which, from the point of view of superficial semblances of images, may be highly dissimilar.

8.2.2. Functional characteristics of coronary arteries

The automatic understanding of 3D images of coronary arteries is the subject of AI research, and as such it is present in the chapter. However, to speak of the understanding of morphological changes in an organ, one must first become acquainted with the organ as such. Obviously, the comments made here are no more than an abstract of an abstract of the vast repository of medical knowledge on coronary arteries that has been gathered. Let the facts that the oxygen and nutrient supply for the heart muscle as well as the removal of final products of metabolism and carbon dioxide is performed through coronary circulation [24] bear witness to the major importance of the correct function of the coronary system – and the advisability of analyzing these anatomic structures in a system of 3D presentation – for the life and well-being of patients. Individual branches of coronary arteries are situated coil-like on the heart's surface so as not to cause increased flow resistance during the contraction and relaxation phases; they supply blood to defined areas of the heart, taking only minor branches to the aorta and the pulmonary trunk [24]. As the layout of the arteries on the diaphragmatic surface of the heart muscle may differ in its shape, three basic types of distribution of these arteries can be distinguished.

The first type is most widespread, and in 60–70% of cases it features a balanced distribution of arteries, with none being dominant. In the second type, the circumflex branch of the left coronary artery is highly retarded while the right coronary artery is highly developed and is the main supplier of blood to the posterior surface of the left ventricle. Such a situation is present in 20–24% of cases on the average, with a variety of intermediate forms possible. In the third type, present in 10–14% cases, the right coronary artery is strongly retarded, while the posterior surface of the right ventricle is vascularized by the left coronary artery, whose anterior interventricular branch may additionally reach the diaphragmatic surface [24]. This shows what difficulties may arise due to the lack of universal standards to allow unambiguous representations of such vessels.

In the case of the sternocostal surface, there are no significant variations of coronary arteries, with the exception of the variations in the anterior interventricular branches, which may be divided into two branches of similar thickness, both in its initial and final section [29].

Besides the variations in the location of the arteries, tasks of constructing semantic representations for spatial visualization of such arteries must account for the possible morphological changes, e.g. in the form of stenoses in their lumen, which attest to progressing pathological processes and lead to coronary diseases.

The coronary art disease, as well as the angina pectoris to which it leads, is usually caused by the development of sclerotic changes which bring about the narrowing of the arteries. This in turn may result in the impairment of arterialized blood flow into a given area of the heart muscle. If one of the major branches of the coronary vessels is suddenly closed, the access of blood is stopped up entirely, and a myocardial infarction occurs in the place not supplied with arterialized blood, and this part of the muscle undergoes necrosis (i.e. dies). Should, however, the obstructions of the flow be less severe or sudden, temporary alterations of heart functions, frequently connected with acute pains (the so-called angina pectoris or stenocardia) may occur, yet they may not be so severe or lethal [24]. Angina pectoris may continue in a stable form with characteristic attacks occurring with foreseeable regularity, in most cases after physical effort or stress, or in its unstable form, whose course may be hard to forecast. Characteristic for it are recurrent and frequently unexpected pains that may occur even at small effort levels or during rest.

The changes listed above are diagnosed to a great extent through a range of specialist methods. The key element of the diagnostic examinations of the heart performed with methods including the angiography of coronary arteries, helical CT scanning, and IVUS are a number of complex algorithms focused on the acquisition and pre-processing of such images [3]. All these examinations are complementary, which provides the diagnostician with vast amounts of information that allows him/her to formulate the proposals of the appropriate diagnosis and to reconstruct information about the structure of coronary vessels. As concerns computer-assisted methods of 3D structure rendering, it is possible to perform visualization of the 3D spatial structure [3]. Application of such methods makes it possible to obtain diagnostic material containing crucial information on the presence and/or advancement of lesions characteristic for certain medical conditions. Most unfortunately, no computer-assisted systems offering automatic interpretation comparable to that conducted by the specialist's keen eye have as yet been built. For that reason, the chapter in its further part describes the manner of developing the linguistic semantic representation of the spatial structure of coronary vessels showing certain pathological changes and their analysis with the use of cognitive methods of image understanding. Thanks to such a description, it will later be possible to support interpretative tasks and define the semantics of actual pathologies.

8.2.3. Graph-based formalisms in the semantic description of coronary vessels

This chapter presents the manner of developing semantic models for the spatial reconstruction of the heart's coronary vessels.

8.2.3.1. Characteristics of the image data

To allow the introduction of linguistic formalisms in the form of a graph-based image grammar that allows finding the stenoses in main arteries or their ramifications and, at the same time, quantifying the lesions discovered, several visualization sequences were performed for the arteries in the DICOM format. Such sequences were obtained for various patients during diagnostic examinations of the heart conducted with tomographic angiography. Such visualizations give a very clear presentation of all morphological changes of individual sections of arteries in any plane. Furthermore, they allow the spatial rendering of coronary vessels to be performed. The examples of a spatial reconstruction of the heart's coronary vessels shown in Fig. 8.9 present the vessels without the accompanying muscle tissue of the heart. Such a reconstruction was obtained from the coronarography images acquired during a diagnostic examination with a helical CT scanner with 64 detectors. It presents the main arteries together with the main minor vessels and a stenosis in the lateral branch and in the initial section of right coronary artery. The structures displayed in this manner will be described with the use of graph-based grammars – constituents of a graph-based language defining their proper, spatial topology.

8.2.3.2. A graph-based description of coronary arteries

The proper graph-based grammar describing these structures was defined so that the individual branches of the graph in the description provided identify all start and end points of coronary vessels and all bifurcations or transitions of main vessels into lower-level ones. The graph-based structure thus developed will constitute the elements of the language for defining the spatial topology and the correct vascularization of the heart muscle together with the potential morphological changes (Fig. 8.9).

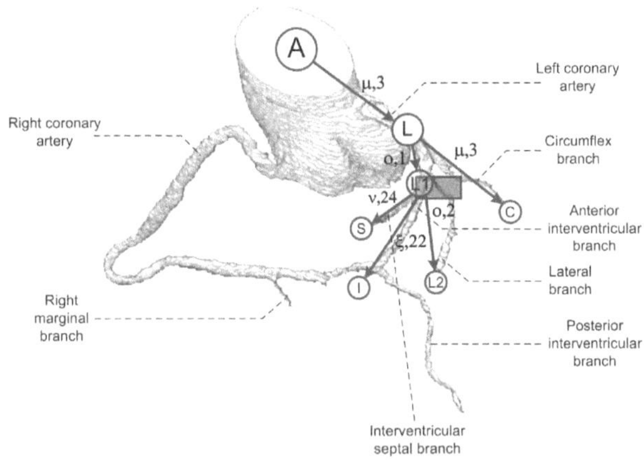

Fig. 8.9.A. The spatial labeling of coronary arteries and defining relations occurring between them for the left coronary artery. The grey rectangle marks the place of a major stenosis in a coronary arterys

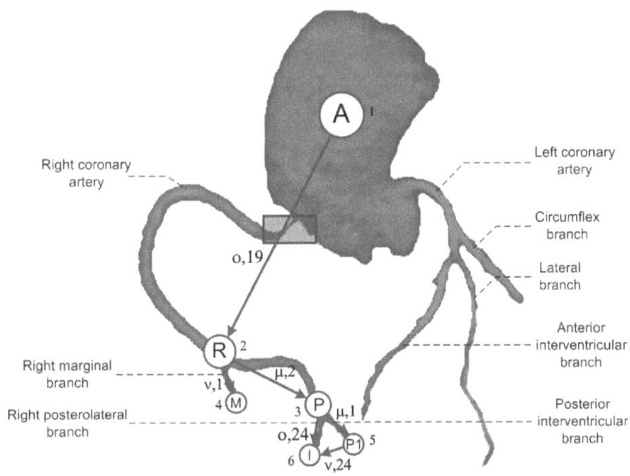

Fig. 8.9.B. The spatial labeling of coronary arteries and defining relations occurring between them for the right coronary artery. The grey rectangle marks the place of a major stenosis in a coronary artery

In practice, the mutual spatial relations that may occur between elements of the vascular structure represented in the form of a graph describe a set of edge labels. Elements of the set are defined by the introduction of appropriate spatial relations:

– vertical, defined by the $\{\alpha, \beta, \ldots, \lambda\}$ set of labels, and

– horizontal, defined by the {1, 2,..., 24} set of labels on the hypothetical sphere surrounding the heart muscle. These labels designate individual sections, each with the angular span of 15°.

Next, for labels defined in this manner, edge terminal labels are assigned to each of the bifurcations marked by the start and end points of appropriate coronary artery sections, depending on the situation of sections of the arteries. Once these relations have been taken into account and node labels of the artery-spanning graph have been entered, it is possible to develop a linguistic description for the purpose of defining the semantics of the lesions looked for and the recognition of pathologic stenoses. This *inter alia* allows for conducting a computer-supported analysis of the rendered structure, aimed at the automatic detection of locations of stenoses, the degree of narrowing and also its type (concentric or eccentric). Such a representation provides a concise and unambiguous description of all the elements of vascular structure in the form of a semantic record. Places where lesions are present are tracked during the constituent analysis of the graph-based representations analyzed, made with the edNLC type grammar. Such an analysis refers to the spatial representation of coronary vessels acquired due to the description developed with the application of IE graphs, a subclass of directed and edge-labeled directed graphs (EDG).

The formal definition of the edNLC type grammar is presented in Chapter 7. It is worth noting that this grammar class is provided with highly efficient syntax analyzers for parsing in multinominal time [54].

To define the places where vessel pathologies occur, a following grammar has been proposed in the graph of coronary arteries presented in Fig. 8.9.A.

$$G_{edNLC} = (\Sigma, \Delta, \Gamma, P, Z), \text{ where:}$$

– $\Sigma = \Sigma_N \cup \Sigma_T$ and is a set of both terminal and non-terminal node labels describing the examined graphs. These labels denote additional nodes in the graphs that are entered as temporary during the syntax analysis or while deriving the representation of a new coronary vascularization.
– $\Delta = \Sigma_T =$ {left coronary artery, anterior interventricular branch, circumflex branch, lateral branch, interventricular septal branch} – a set of terminal node labels describe the terminal elements of the modeled structure of the heart's vessels. (presented also in Fig. 8.9.A).
– $\Sigma_N =$ {A, B, C, D, E, I, L, L1, L2, S} is a set of non-terminal node labels.
– $\Gamma = \{\mu,3;\ \nu,24;\ \xi,22;\ o,1;\ o,2\}$ is a finite, non-empty set of edge labels. This set makes it possible to define spatial relations occurring between the individual sections approximating the recognized vessels.
– Z = {B} is the original starting graph, which is used to begin the process of generation of all graph-based forms for coronary arteries.
– P is a finite set of productions recorded in a parenthesis-based form and with the use of diagrammatic graph-based notation (Fig. 8.10).

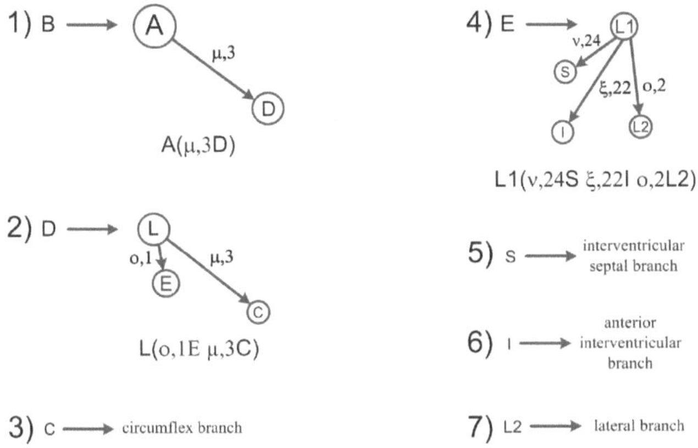

Fig. 8.10. Production set for the G_{edNLC} grammar

To define the location where the vessel pathology is present in the graph of coronary arteries in Fig. 8.9.B, the following grammar is proposed.

$$G_{edNLC} = (\Sigma, \Delta, \Gamma, P, Z), \text{ where:}$$

- $\Sigma = \Sigma_N \cup \Sigma_T$ and is a set of both terminal and non-terminal node labels describing the examined graphs and defined as follows.
- $\Delta = \Sigma_T =$ {right coronary artery, right marginal branch, right posterolateral branch, posterior interventricular branch} – a set of terminal node labels (presented also in Fig. 8.9.B).
- $\Sigma_N =$ {A, B, C, I, M, P, P1, R} is a set of non-terminal node labels.
- $\Gamma = \{\mu,1;\ \mu,2;\ \nu,1;\ \nu,24;\ o,19;\ o,24\}$ is a set of labels describing edges of the graph.
- Z = {A} is the original starting graph.
- P – is a finite set of productions recorded in the graph-based form and presented in Fig. 8.10

It is worth mentioning that inference in a graph-based grammar of the $G_{edNLC} = (\Sigma, \Delta, \Gamma, P, Z)$ type is defined recurrently in accordance with the following principles:

1. Generation begins with the graph ***g*** composed of a single node with the label ***Z***.
2. Then if in ***g*** there exists a non-terminal node ***n*** labeled with the symbol ***l*** from the set of node labels Σ, and the (l, D, C) triad belongs to the production set defined in the grammar, then the node ***n*** is replaced by a defined EDG-class graph ***D***. The embedding transformation $C : \Gamma \times \{\text{in, out}\} \rightarrow 2^{\Sigma\times\Sigma\times\Gamma\times\{\text{in, out}\}}$ is applied here in the following manner. Having assumed the existence of a production with the embedding transformation defined as (a, c, y, out)∈C(x, in), the edge labeled by ***x***, which enters the non-terminal node ***n***, is replaced by an edge labeled as ***y***, leaving the node ***a*** of the defined graph ***D*** and connecting it to the node labeled with the symbol ***c*** of the output graph.

As the edNLC-class grammar derived above allows a spatial analysis of the structure described with IE graphs, quoting the formal definition of such structures is justified.

Definition 8.1. The name of an IE graph (indexed edge-unambiguous) is applied to the system [51]:

$$H = (V, E, \Sigma, \Gamma, \varphi), \text{ where:}$$

- V is a finite, non-empty set of graph nodes with unambiguously assigned indices,
- Σ is a finite, non-empty set of node labels,
- Γ is a finite, non-empty set of edge labels,
- E is a set of graph edges in the form of (v, λ, w), where $v, w \in V$, $\lambda \in \Gamma$ and the index v is smaller than the index w,
- $\varphi : V \rightarrow \Sigma$ – the function of node labeling.

The IE graph presented in Fig. 8.11 together with the characteristic description of the nodes present therein may be used to describe the selected sections of the coronary vessels presented in the Fig. 8.9.B.

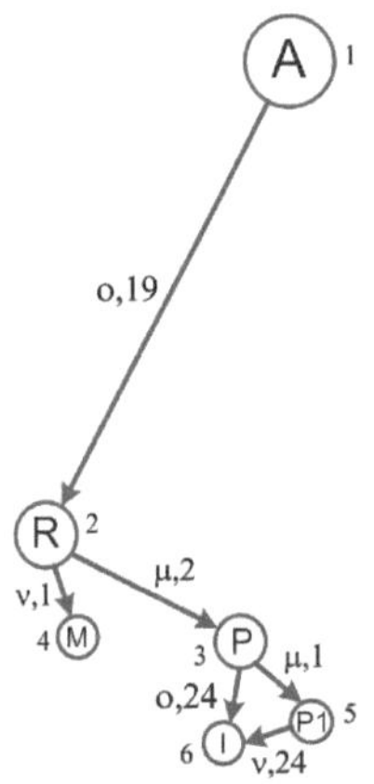

A_1	R_2	P_3	M_4	Pl_5	I_6
1	2	2	0	1	0
o,19	μ,2 ν,1	μ,1 o,24	-	ν,24	-
2	3 4	5 6	-	6	-

Fig. 8.11. A representation of the spatial reconstruction of coronary vessels using an IE graph together with a vertex characteristic description

For the graph-based grammar introduced earlier, the set of deriving rules in the form of IE graphs, which allow for deriving the spatial representation if the right coronary artery described in Fig. 8.9.B is presented in Fig. 8.12.

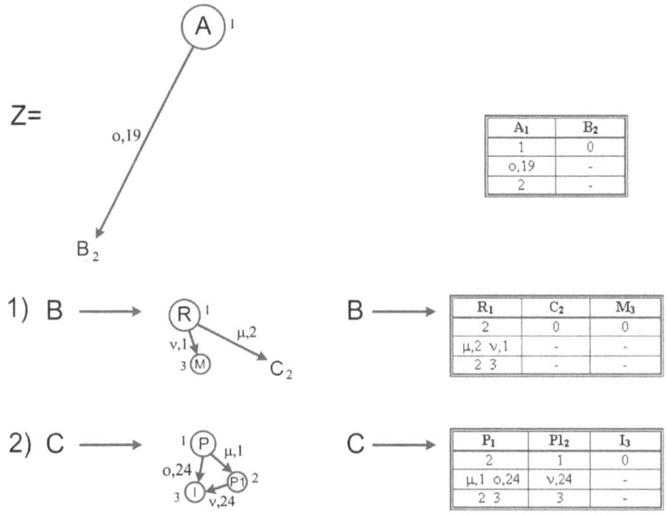

Fig. 8.12. A set of productions in the form of IE graphs deriving the structure of coronary vessels together with the vertex characteristic description

8.2.3.3. A semantic analysis of the coronary structure

After a final description of the image using the grammar presented above, we must implement syntax analyzers which conduct the cognitive resonance analysis. This is obviously the most difficult part of the whole task, especially for the graph and tree grammars. During cognitive resonance, the analyzer must generate a semantic description of the image under consideration, which must have been verified with grammar rules. Such a verification is performed by the parser of the grammar used. Hypothesis generation is connected with the use of a selected production (mappings included into the formal description of the grammar). The hypothesis is verified by incessantly comparing selected features of coronary vessels with some expectations taken from the source of knowledge represented in grammar rules. The details of a parsing algorithm for edNLC graph grammars can be found in [54].

Apart from the straight syntax analysis of the input graph sequence, syntax analyzers are capable of performing semantic actions assigned to individual productions (grammar rules). This allows for generating certain values or information which is the result of the syntactic analysis performed. Every time the parser uses one of productions for generation the final graph, simultaneously it performs a semantic action assigned to it. Usually the objective of such an action is to compute the semantic value of the final graph representation on the basis of semantic values of individual components of this expression.

It is worth noting that it is the semantic analysis that plays a key role in computer-aided understanding of semantic image contents. Apart from the knowledge and expectations defined by grammar rules and the productions introduced, it is these very semantic actions that allow one to compute the morphometric parameters of the analyzed lesions which need to be calculated. Owing to the use of additional knowledge on the form, their location in a given vessel and the advancement stage (the degree of lumen stricture), it is possible to draw conclusions about the significance of the case analyzed.

8.2.4. Selected results

As the research conducted proves, by applying the formalisms and graph-based grammars presented in the study, it is possible to develop semantic descriptions and to spatially model the morphology of coronary vessels as well as to discover symptoms of ischemia in them. Such lesions are discovered by determining the place of their occurrence, i.e. be defining the position of the vessel and the degree of the stenosis of the artery lumen, and by the designation of morphometric parameters defining its scope and type (eccentric or concentric). One central element of the syntactic and semantic analysis consists in parsing which, in the case of a structural analysis of the representations developed, automatically provides (thanks to the use of semantic actions and procedures) complete information defining the spatial topology of the graph in question and describing the coronary vessels together with their individual constituents. Subsequently, that information is used for the structural and semantic analysis of individual sections of arteries, which are defined by terminal node and edge labels. This allows for the precise definition of morphological irregularities in the vessels examined that may be present in the form of various stenoses [29]. All the information mentioned here makes it possible to develop a semantic record containing the semantic description of the structure in question. Such descriptions may provide a certain type of indexing keys that allow the data to be archived and found (in the form of 3D visualizations) using information about the pathological conditions present. Due to the small set of test data (covering a dozen elements) the results achieved are highly promising. Such efficiency, however, is also the result of the high generalization properties of the formalisms applied.

The image set of recognition data, which has been used to determine the efficiency of the correct recognition of the size of stenoses in coronary arteries in percentage terms, included 16 different spatial reconstructions obtained for patients with heart diseases (mostly ischemia). In this set, we considered image sequences of patients previously analyzed at the stage of the grammar construction and the recognizing analyzer. In order to avoid analyzing identical reconstructions, we selected separate images occurring after a slight position rotation (a different projection) compared to the ones used originally (from spatial helical CT scans). The remaining images in the test data had been obtained for a new group of patients. The objective of the analysis of this data was to determine the efficiency of the correct recognition of artery stenoses, expressed in percentages, and to determine their size with the use of the grammar introduced. On the image data tested, the efficiency of recognition amounted to 85%. The efficiency of recognition is equal to the percentage of the accurately recognized and measured vessel stenoses compared to the total number of images analyzed in the test. The recognition itself meant locating and defining the type of stenosis, e.g. concentric or eccentric.

The results achieved also prove that, by applying the described type of grammar, allowing the semantic interpretation of the spatial reconstruction of coronary vessels, it is possible to analyze the correct morphology of individual sections of arteries and their branches. This greatly extends the scope of applying AI methodologies for computer-assisted methods of understanding diagnostic images and defining the medical significance of pathologies present in them.

Certain questions were not resolved by the research conducted, namely the question of the automatic selection of the proper projection of coronary vessels in a manner allowing the most unambiguous visualization of the pathologies present. Though at this stage there is no automatic procedure for searching for such a projection, the question remains the subject of further research on the methods presented. Another problem is the question of automating the process of generating new grammars for cases not accounted for in the existent language. The processes of developing new grammars and augmenting already existing ones with new description rules represent another subject followed by the authors.

When characterizing the proposed approach, it is worth noting that the fundamental difference between syntactic methods and widely applied methods, included the group of minimal distance methods [18] (e.g. template matching), is that syntax analyzers can recognize lesions in a more general manner i.e. due to the lack of an ideal pattern. To diagnose pathological lesions in the morphology of analyzed organs one cannot determine a full and finite didactic set, which would include all possible forms of pathologies listed. This is an obvious consequence of the fact that every patient is unique due to the occurrence of idiosyncratic anatomical differences. It is therefore impossible to provide a universal pattern in the form of one reconstruction of coronary arteries specifying a model or standard shape of healthy or normal vessels.

Due to the fact that in medical image analysis there are difficulties with supplying a representative and at the same time universal model, it is not possible to use algorithms and computer-aided learning methods on an exclusive basis [26]. Nor is it possible to apply measurement methods of the similarity or differentiation of examined images in order to analyze these structures in an unequivocal manner. This means that, in this case, it is necessary to use intelligent image recognition methods which not only enable processing and detecting simple objects, but also facilitate a wider semantic analysis and the determination of features of extremely complex structures like coronary arteries and their reconstructions.

8.2.5. Conclusions concerning the semantic analysis of coronary artery images

The approach to the cognitive interpretation of spatial visualizations of coronary vessels presented in this study represents a significant innovation among the tasks of 3D computer-assisted medical diagnostics. This is because applying graph-based image languages in the spatial modeling of coronary structures makes it possible to define the semantics of pathological changes present in them. The application of such formalisms also offers vast opportunities to focus interpretation tasks on the performance of the automatic analysis and detection of actual morphological irregularities in a perceptive manner, which inspires the development of cognitive information systems based on graph-based image languages.

Such methods are of profound significance as they allow not only for the discovery of lesions but also for the definition of their semantics, which – in the case of medical diagnostic images – may lead to computer-assisted 'understanding' of their medical significance and also to fine-tuning the optimum therapeutic options in the future. It is worth noting the huge progress of medical engineering in the field of intelligent information systems and the great similarity between the operation of the presented model of structural analysis and the interpretative cognitive procedures taking place in the human mind. Despite the often complex process of grammar-based reasoning, syntactic methods of image recognition making use of graph-based image languages in the analysis of the spatial structure of the heart vascularization provide nearly all the information for the description of morphological changes in coronary vessels. Such information may be useful in tasks of both diagnostic and therapeutic nature as well as in the tasks of context-sensitive semantic searches for specific visualization cases.

8.3. Concluding remarks

In this chapter we showed that the methodology of the linguistic description of complex images and the automatic understanding of their substantive (diagnostic) content can be more universal than predicted by scientists right after that new technology was defined. Taking into account that the core idea of automatic understanding of images is achieved during the parsing process connected with the use of the cognitive resonance paradigm, we showed in this chapter (and in some papers printed before this book was written) that the same methodology can be extended to cover new classes of medical images.

The methodology under consideration was previously used for the semantic analysis of 2D medical images which contained **one object** of interest only (e.g. the pancreatic duct, the spinal cord or the ureter). The first part of this chapter shows how to overcome these limitations and use the developed methodology for the analysis and the semantic description of multi-object images. The analysis and also the understanding of this type of medical images is more complicated because one image contains many morphological elements, which must be assessed not only on the basis of their own (individual) shapes, but also on the basis of their connections and spatial relations. The second part of this chapter shows how to extend methods used during the semantic analysis of 2D images for the semantic interpretation of 3D images.

On the basis of results presented in this chapter and taking into account the yet unpublished results of current research, we can stress that the methodology of automatic understanding of medical images can be used for more complicated tasks than was previously predicted. It has not been proven yet, but we can predict and expect that such a methodology can be properly adapted to almost all medical images. The only assumption is that it is possible to describe the most important features of the considered images in terms of a particular language. If we can define the language which can describe the most important substantive features of the analyzed images, then we can also describe the grammar for this language. When the proposed grammar can include not only a formal description of the image structure, but also a semantic description of the substantive meaning of particular morphological forms, we can also develop an effective tool for performing the cognitive resonance during the parsing process. Currently, this tool has to be developed separately for every particular medical problem on the basis of the analysis of images taken into account as well as on the basis of the medical knowledge collected from experts. However, we expect that one of the directions in which the proposed methods will be developed and improved will be to unify the methodology and the forming methods for the automatic generation of languages and grammars using a specified learning process.

References

1. Albus JS, Meystel AM (2001) Engineering of Mind: An Introduction to the Science of Intelligent Systems. Willey
2. Bakal CW, Silberzweig JE, Cynamon J, Sprayregen S (2002) Vascular and Interventional Radiology: Principles and Practice. Thieme, Stuttgart
3. Bankman I (ed) (2002) Handbook of Medical Imaging: Processing and Analysis. Academic Press, San Diego
4. Block B (2004) Color Atlas of Ultrasound Anatomy. Thieme, Stuttgart
5. Bluth EI, Benson C, Ralls PW, Siegel MJ (2000) Ultrasound-A Practical Approach to Clinical Problems. Thieme, Stuttgart
6. Bodzioch S (2006) Automatic recognition of selected gallbladder diseases basing on analyzing of the static ultrasonographic images. Ph. D. Thesis, AGH University of Science an d Technology, Krakow
7. Bodzioch S (2006) Automated detecting symptoms of selected gallbladder illness based on a static ultrasound images analysis. Bio-Algorithms and Med-Systems 2(3):33-42
8. Boliek M, Zandi A (1995) CREW: lossless/lossy image compression: contribution to ISO/IEC JTC 1.29.12. ISO Working Document ISO/IEC JTC1/SC29/WG1 N196
9. Burgener FA, Kormano M (1997) Bone and Joint Disorders. Thieme, Stuttgart
10. Burgener FA, Meyers SP, Tan R. (2001) Differential diagnosis in Magnetic Resonance Imaging. Thieme, Stuttgart
11. Carpentieri B, Weinberger MJ, Seroussi G (2000) Lossless Compression of Continuous Tone Images
12. Christopoulos C, Skodras A, Ebrahimi T (2000) The JPEG2000 Still Image Coding System an Overview. IEEE Transactions on Consumer Electronics 46(4)
13. Clunie DA (2000) Losseless compression of grayscale medical images – effectiveness of traditional and state of the art approaches
14. Davis LS (2001) Foundations of image understanding. Kluwer
15. Denecker K, Van Overloop J, Lemahieu I (1997) An experimental comparison of several lossless image coders for medical images. Proc. Of the Data Compression Industry Workshop, Snowbird, Utah, USA
16. Digital Imaging and Communications in Medicine (DICOM). National Electrical Manufacturers Association, 1300 N. 17th Street, Rosslyn, Virginia 22209 USA. 2001
17. Donohoe KJ, Van den Abbeele AD (2000) Teaching Atlas of Nuclear Medicine. Thieme, Stuttgart
18. Duda RO, Hart PE, Stork DG (2001) Pattern classifications. 2nd Ed, Willey
19. Flasiński M (1993) On the parsing of deterministic graph languages for syntactic pattern recognition. Pattern Recognition 26:1-16
20. Higgins WE, Karwoski RA, Ritman EL, Spyra WJ (1996) System for analyzing true three-dimensional angiograms. IEEE Trans. Med. Imag. 15:377-385
21. Higgins WE, Reinhardt JM (2000) Cardiac image processing, in Handbook of Video and Image Processing, ed.A. Bovik, Academic Press, San-Diego
22. Hoffman KR, Sen A, Li Lan (2000) A system for determination of 3D vessel tree centerlines from biplane images. The International Journal of Cardiac Imaging 16:315-330
23. Janssens D, Rozenberg G, Verraedt R (1982) On sequential and parallel node-rewriting graph grammars. Computer Graphics and Image Processing 18:279-304
24. Khan MG (1996) Heart Disease Diagnosis and Therapy.Williams & Wilkins, Baltimore
25. Lin EC, Alavi A (2006) PET and PET/CT-A Clinical Guide. Thieme, Stuttgart
26. Meyer-Base A (2004) Pattern Recognition for Medical Imaging. Elsevier Academic
27. Mikrut Z (1996) A Method of Linear Star-Sections Applied for Object Separation in ERCP Images. Proceedings of International Conference on Image Processing 363-366
28. Najarian K, Splinter R (2006) Biomedical Signal and Image Processing. CRC
29. Netter FH, Colacino S (1998) Atlas of Human Anatomy. Novartis Medical Education

30. Ogiela L, Tadeusiewicz R, Ogiela MR (2006) Cognitive Analysis In Diagnostic DSS-Type IT Systems. LNAI 4029:962-971
31. Ogiela L, Tadeusiewicz R, Ogiela MR (2006) Cognitive Approach to Visual Data Interpretation in Medical Information and Recognition Systems. LNCS 4153:244-250
32. Ogiela L, Tadeusiewicz R, Ogiela MR (2006) Graph-Based Structural Data Mining in Cognitive Pattern Interpretation. LNAI 4201:349-350
33. Ogiela L, Tadeusiewicz R, Ogiela MR (2006) Cognitive Computing in Intelligent Medical Pattern Recognition Systems. LNCIS 344:851-856
34. Ogiela MR (1998) Languages of shape feature description and syntactic methods for recognition of morphological changes of organs in analysis of selected X-ray images. SPIE Vol. 3338:1295-1305
35. Ogiela MR (2007) Automatic understanding of medical images based on grammar approach. In IEEE Proceedings: IEEE Catalog Number: 07EX1676C ISBN: 1-4244-0965-9 Library of Congress: 2007920354, CD paper No 1569030913.pdf, pp.1-4
36. Ogiela MR, Tadeusiewicz R (2000) Syntactic pattern recognition for X-ray diagnosis of pancreatic cancer. IEEE ENGINEERING IN MEDICINE AND BIOLOGY MAGAZINE, 19(6):94-105
37. Ogiela MR, Tadeusiewicz R (2003) Cognitive Vision Systems in Medical Applications. LNAI 2871:116-123
38. Ogiela MR, Tadeusiewicz R (2004) Picture Languages in Intelligent Retrieval of Visual Data Semantic Information. LNAI 3336:389-396
39. Ogiela MR, Tadeusiewicz R (2005) Nonlinear Processing and Semantic Content Analysis in Medical Imaging – A Cognitive Approach. IEEE Transactions on Instrumentation and Measurement, 54(6):2149-2155
40. Ogiela MR, Tadeusiewicz R (2005) Picture Languages in Medical Pattern Knowledge Representation and Understanding. LNAI 3558:442-447
41. Ogiela MR, Tadeusiewicz R (2005) Picture Languages in Machine Understanding of Medical Visualization. Machine Graphics and Vision 14(1):71-82
42. Ogiela MR, Tadeusiewicz R (2005) Intelligent Recognition in Medical Pattern Understanding and Cognitive Analysis. In Muhammad Sarfraz (ed), Computer-Aided Intelligent Recognition Techniques and Applications, John Wiley & Sons, 257-274
43. Ogiela MR, Tadeusiewicz R, Ogiela L (2006) Image Languages in Intelligent Radiological Palm Diagnostics. Pattern Recognition 39:2157-2165
44. Ogiela MR, Tadeusiewicz R, Trzupek M (2007) Graph-based semantic description in medical knowledge representation and 3D coronary vessels recognition. LNCS, 4611:1079-1088
45. Pavlidis T (1982) Algorithms for Graphics and Image Processing. Computer Science Press, Rockville
46. Pietka E et al (2001) Computer-Assisted Bone Age Assessment: Image Preprocessing and Epiphyseal/Metahyseal ROI Extraction. IEEE Trans. On Medical Imaging, 20(8):715-729
47. Pratt WK (2007) Digital Image Processing 4th ed. Wiley & Sons, Hoboken, New Jersey
48. Ritter GX, Wilson JN (1996) Computer Vision Algorithms in Image Algebra. CRC Press, Inc., Boca Raton
49. Shi QY, Fu KS (1983) Parsing and translation of attributed expansive graph languages for scene analysis. IEEE Trans. PAMI 5:472-483
50. Skomorowski M (1998) Parsing of random graphs for scene analysis. Machine GRAPHICS & VISION 7:313-323
51. Skomorowski M (2000) A Syntactic-Statistical Approach to Recognition of Distorted Patterns. Jagiellonian University, Krakow (in Polish)
52. Sonka M, Fitzpatrick JM (2000) Medical Imaging, Vol. 2. Medical Image processing and Analysis. SPIE PRESS
53. Starck JL, Murtagh F, Candès EJ, Donoho DL (2003) Gray and Color Image Contrast Enhancement by the Curvelet Transform. IEEE Trans on Image Proc. 12(6)
54. Tadeusiewicz R, Flasiński M (1991) Pattern Recognition, Warsaw (in Polish)

55. Tadeusiewicz R, Ogiela MR (2004) Medical Image Understanding Technology, Springer, Berlin-Heidelberg
56. Tadeusiewicz R, Ogiela MR (2004) The new concept in computer vision: automatic understanding of the images. LNAI 3070:133-144
57. Tadeusiewicz R, Ogiela MR (2005) Picture Languages in Automatic Radiological Palm Interpretation. International Journal of Applied Mathematics and Computer Science 15(2):305-312
58. Tadeusiewicz R, Ogiela MR (2006) New Results Obtained Using the Medical Images Automatic Understanding Technologies. In Piętka E, Łęski J, Franiel S (eds) Medical Informatics & Technologies, Proceedings of the XI International Conference, MIT 2006, I-3 – I-15
59. Tadeusiewicz R, Ogiela MR (2006) Automatic Image Understanding- A New Paradigm for Intelligent Medical Image Analysis. BIO-ALGORITHMS AND MED-SYSTEMS 2(3):5-11
60. Tadeusiewicz R, Ogiela MR (2007) Why Automatic Understanding?. LNCS 4432:477- 491
61. Tadeusiewicz R, Ogiela MR, Ogiela L(2007) A New Approach to the Computer Support of Strategic Decision Making in Enterprises by Means of a New Class of Understanding Based Management Support Systems. In Saeed K, Abraham A, Mosdorf R (eds) IEEE Computer Society, 2007, pp. 9-13
62. Taubman D (2000) High Performance Scalable Image Compression With EBCOT. IEEE Trans. Image Processing 9(7)
63. Wang Z, Bovik AC, Sheikh HR, Simoncelli EP (2004) Image quality assessment: from error visibility to structural similarity. IEEE Trans. on Image Processing 13(4):600–612
64. Weinberger MJ, Seroussi G, Sapiro G (2000) The LOCO-I lossless image compression algorithm: Principles and standardization into JPEG-LS. IEEE Trans. Image Processing 9(8)
65. Wu X (1997) Efficient Lossless Compression of Continuous-tone Images via Context Selection and Quantization. IEEE Trans. on Image Processing

Index

MIX
Papier aus verantwortungsvollen Quellen
Paper from responsible sources
FSC® C105338

If you have any concerns about our products,
you can contact us on
ProductSafety@springernature.com

In case Publisher is established outside the EU,
the EU authorized representative is:
Springer Nature Customer Service Center GmbH
Europaplatz 3, 69115 Heidelberg, Germany

Printed by Libri Plureos GmbH
in Hamburg, Germany